ADHD
Unpacked

ADHD
Unpacked

Everything you need to know to survive and thrive as an adult with ADHD

Alex Conner & James Brown

TONIC

LONDON · OXFORD · NEW YORK · NEW DELHI · SYDNEY

BLOOMSBURY TONIC
Bloomsbury Publishing Plc
50 Bedford Square, London, WC1B 3DP, UK
Bloomsbury Publishing Ireland Limited,
29 Earlsfort Terrace, Dublin 2, D02 AY28, Ireland

BLOOMSBURY, BLOOMSBURY TONIC and the Tonic logo are trademarks
of Bloomsbury Publishing Plc

First published in Great Britain 2025

Copyright © Alex Conner and James Brown, 2025

Alex Conner and James Brown are identified as the authors of this work in
accordance with the Copyright, Designs and Patents Act 1988.

All rights reserved. No part of this publication may be: i) reproduced or
transmitted in any form, electronic or mechanical, including photocopying,
recording or by means of any information storage or retrieval system without
prior permission in writing from the publishers; or ii) used or reproduced in
any way for the training, development or operation of artificial intelligence (AI)
technologies, including generative AI technologies. The rights holders expressly
reserve this publication from the text and data mining exception as per Article
4(3) of the Digital Single Market Directive (EU) 2019/790

Bloomsbury Publishing Plc does not have any control over, or responsibility
for, any third-party websites referred to in this book. All internet addresses given
in this book were correct at the time of going to press. The author and publisher
regret any inconvenience caused if addresses have changed or sites have
ceased to exist, but can accept no responsibility for any such changes

A catalogue record for this book is available from the British Library

ISBN: TPB: 978-1-5266-7936-9; eBook: 978-1-5266-7935-2;
ePDF: 978-1-5266-7934-5

2 4 6 8 10 9 7 5 3 1

Typeset by Ed Pickford

Printed and bound in Great Britain by Clays Ltd, Elcograf S.p.A.

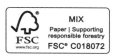

To find out more about our authors and books visit www.bloomsbury.com
and sign up for our newsletters

For product safety related questions contact
productsafety@bloomsbury.com

This book v   out the magical creature that is Mrs Au.   en me a second life. I also dedicate this book to Robert from Kidderminster.

James Brown

I learned to love laughter, science and languages from my mum and dad and brothers. I grew up in a safe place, so I was able to meet and marry someone perfect for me and to have a healthy, safe and loving family of my own. This book is dedicated to the family that raised me and the family I raised. I love you all.

Alex Conner

Contents

	Prologue	1
1	What is ADHD?	15
2	What causes ADHD?	31
3	ADHD and the brain	49
4	Myth-understandings!	61
5	ADHD isn't a superpower for everybody	81
6	ADHD diagnosis	91
7	ADHD treatment	117
8	Pay attention!	135
9	Sit still and don't interrupt!	155
10	Reward and ADHD	167
11	Emotions and rejection in ADHD	179
12	Executive functions and ADHD	201
13	Sex, relationships and ADHD	213
14	ADHD & the 4 Ps: prioritisation, procrastination, perfectionism and productivity	229
15	ADHD+: comorbidities	245
16	How to navigate a neurotypical world	255
	References	269
	Acknowledgements	279

Prologue

Thanks for picking up this book. We really hope you like it and feel that you know more about ADHD in adults after reading it. More importantly, we hope this book makes you feel less alone – or less different – if you have (or suspect you have) ADHD.

We are very fortunate to be part of a huge and supportive network of adults with ADHD. Before we tell you more about ADHD, we want to explain how we got here.

We are probably best known for a podcast called 'The ADHD Adults', which we release weekly with the inimitable Mrs AuDHD. Our podcast tries to make sense of all the ADHD science and evidence, comparing it with our lived experiences, and deals with a lot of the stigma, myths and misunderstandings out there on the internet. We have also founded a small charity called ADHDadultUK, which is designed for anyone with an interest in the success and support of adults with ADHD.

As well as working together on the podcast and charity, we have been scientists and friends for a long time. To explain our partnership and why we aim to support the ADHD

James's story

My journey to get a diagnosis of ADHD wasn't particularly typical, if there is such a thing. If I look back long enough, I can remember at some point in the early 1980s, living in rural Shropshire, the family doctor said to my mum, 'Don't worry, Mrs Brown, he's hyperactive, but he'll grow out of it.' This was clearly not true – the 'he'll grow out of it' part, that is.

As a child, I was very overly hyperactive, and this has never really gone away. To this day, I can't sit still when I make a phone call, and whenever I visit my mum, I stand and walk around while I talk to her.

I felt different for most of my life. I always felt like I was 'other', especially as a child and teenager. My people-pleasing meant I was often in trouble, getting suspended – and in some cases, even arrested. These things happened because I desperately wanted to appear to be like my friends.

Looking back, I don't think I had the right friends. I was an intelligent child – I had a reading age of twelve when I was seven years old ... In fact, I probably still have a reading age of twelve now, at the ripe age of forty-nine. But most of my school reports stated that I needed to focus more, that I wasn't using my abilities, and that if I 'knuckled down' I could be a success. Obviously I did none of these things,

PROLOGUE

and I now realise that this is because I had undiagnosed ADHD. I also now realise that my self-loathing comes from this time, when I felt alone and different to everyone around me.

The intelligence I had didn't translate into academic performance. Despite studying hard to achieve a PhD and becoming a professor, my grades at school were average and at the time not good enough for university. I initially decided to become a nurse. I was terrible at the job and (looking back now) fortunately broke my spine before I could complete my nursing qualification, which led me to do a degree in biomedical science.

I was always fascinated by biology, and the only book I regularly read as a child was an illustrated encyclopaedia on health and disease. This meant I could tell you what a keloid scar was when I was seven (oddly, this didn't win me friends). This love of biology was the reason I managed to study it to a high level; I found it rewarding to learn more about the human body.

When I was awarded my PhD and became a researcher, I wasn't good at the things most researchers need to be good at, such as actually doing experiments and writing funding applications or scientific papers. Most researchers have one area of speciality, but I had six or seven as I kept jumping from subject to subject as each 'shiny thing' interested me. In a way, it led me to this book.

One day, I had a random phone call from the BBC asking if I would fill in for a scientist who had dropped out of a television programme called *The Truth About Fat*. As the filming didn't go terribly, it was followed by programme after programme, and I soon became a happy science communicator, as opposed to an unhappy scientist.

Around this time, and unexpectedly, my concept of who I was, and why I was different, changed. This story may not be completely true, but the day that Alex was diagnosed with ADHD, he phoned me up and said something like, 'I've just been diagnosed with ADHD and you're way more ADHD than I am!'

At the time, I had just been promoted to senior lecturer in biomedical science and was teaching neurophysiology to students. I am embarrassed to say that I didn't know adults could have ADHD. Like many people, I thought ADHD was just something schoolboys had and that they grew out of it to some degree. After Alex and I had a good chat, I immediately went online and filled in the Adult ADHD self-report scale (ASRS). The response I received suggested very strongly that I had the symptoms of ADHD. I did nothing with this information for several years, and even helped a colleague to get his own diagnosis after telling him that it was likely he had ADHD, before doing anything for myself. In a way, this sums me up: help others – don't help yourself.

There are two main reasons why I didn't pursue a diagnosis. Firstly, I thought I was doing 'well in life'. I had just been promoted, which is often how we measure success. I was a trustee of the world's oldest ageing research organisation and held multiple senior roles within my university. To me, this meant my life was going well. With the power of

PROLOGUE

hindsight, I was struggling though. My mental health was poor, I had little life outside of work, my relationship with Mrs AuDHD (my long-suffering wife) was at times strained, and I was fundamentally unhappy.

The second reason that I didn't consider pursuing an assessment for ADHD was because I was medication hesitant. This may sound ridiculous, but although I have incredibly low self-esteem, to the point of hating myself most of the time, I was worried that taking medication for ADHD would 'change me'. Reading this back, it sounds as absurd as it is.

For me, everything changed during the second national lockdown during the COVID-19 pandemic. Because all university teaching moved online, and all lectures had to be rewritten, rebranded and delivered virtually via a computer in my home office, I ended up working seven days a week, ten hours a day, and worked myself into burnout.

For three months, Alex, Mrs AuDHD and my lovely colleague Eric (who I had suggested should get a diagnosis) repeatedly told me that I needed to get a diagnosis myself and that I was struggling. All I could think of was doing my job, making sure I kept the students and my employer happy, and not stopping until the work was done. At the end of this teaching term, on the very first day that I wasn't working, I collapsed. I was emotionally and physically empty.

I now know that this is burnout, and once the adrenaline that had kept me going for three months had gone, I had nothing left in the tank. This put me into a mental health crisis, which culminated in me sitting on the sofa on Christmas

Day staring at the wall thinking about how much I no longer wanted to exist. It was a turning point. In the new year, I started to investigate how to get an ADHD assessment. As I was already aware that the waiting list was extraordinarily long, I decided to pursue a private assessment, with financial support from my mum.

On 2 February 2021, I was diagnosed with ADHD. Of all the events that have happened in my life, including birthdays, graduations and even my wedding day, this date is probably the most crucial in my life so far. It changed everything.

It enabled me to see all the events that had occurred in my life through a different lens, changing how I viewed my past. Where I had once blamed myself for being 'lazy', 'unreliable' or 'useless', I now understood that there was a reason why these things happened. It also helped me and Mrs AuDHD to look at the issues we had as a couple and to understand that there was a reason why we had them. Finally, it gave me a future.

Two months prior, I didn't see a future for myself. I didn't want a future for myself. I wanted the world to open a James-sized hole and swallow me up. Now I could see that there was a future for me.

Since my diagnosis, and since co-founding the charity ADHDadultUK as well as The ADHD Adults Podcast, my life has purpose. Knowing what I now know about ADHD, after spending pretty much every day learning everything I can about the biology, psychology and neurophysiology of ADHD, and reflecting on my own experiences, I am now able to help other people who have ADHD. When I was diagnosed, that help wasn't available to me.

After my diagnosis, Alex and I chatted and we agreed that there was extraordinarily little out there to help people with ADHD understand themselves, explain ADHD to their partners or colleagues at work, and learn to manage their symptoms beyond very bland and generalised advice. We also agreed that we were going to change this.

I hope that if I am still here in a few years' time that I can look back at that diagnosis, at the way in which it changed not just my life in general, but my career, and that hopefully the work I've done alongside Alex, Mrs AuDHD and others, including this book, has helped people with ADHD. To me, that means everything I have been through – the struggles, the substance abuse issues, the mental health crises, and everything else I struggled with – has been worth it. Even if I have helped just one person, it will all have been worth it.

Alex's story

I was diagnosed with ADHD in my thirties. Later, when I asked my mum if it was obvious with hindsight, she first said no. But then she thought for a minute and said, 'Well, we knew something wasn't right.' This is one of my favourite quotes.

I am one of those people who can be accurately described as 'living with supported, treated and managed ADHD'. I am still a hot mess but it is my mess. I don't think there is a lot in my story that will be completely unfamiliar to people diagnosed as an adult. I wasn't naughty at school (or I wasn't caught) and this put me under the radar. I wasn't shouting or breaking things, and I wasn't rocking any boats either. Instead, I was sad.

Almost every single second of high school felt like a slow and laborious torture of boredom. I was 'fidgety' and 'distracted'. I could never figure out how everyone knew that we had to have our sports clothes or bring a textbook or do homework. It all seemed baffling to me – and my God, was I bored (apart from drama or those incredibly rare moments when we would do an activity in class). I really didn't realise that other people were not actively, cripplingly tortured with feelings of boredom. I assumed everyone felt like that and I was just weak. 'It's just willpower,' I would say to myself. 'A character flaw.' I always knew I was different. But then everyone says that, don't they?

Growing up, my family was (and still is) very 'high energy'. Please note that I would NEVER diagnose other people without their explicit permission. What I am saying is that my family would often use the phrase 'but everyone is like that' for behaviours that (I now realise) are extremely connected with ADHD.

Many of my ADHD symptoms, from hyperactivity to boredom and general 'wildness', were quite normal in my family. I knew it was unusual, but looking back I just assumed that we as a family were the normal ones and most people were a bit dull. I grew up in an ADHD-friendly family, and one of the greatest compliments I can give to my parents and my

PROLOGUE

brothers is that I felt safe at home. I still feel safe with them. Despite their many, MANY personal failings. I had to add that last bit or they would think I was ill.

Away from home was a different story. Even from a very early age, I knew something was wrong with me. I knew I was clever because people tell you that when you are five years old. But I struggled (and still struggle) with some of the basic elements of life, such as sitting still or paying attention. I would get incredibly enthusiastic or ugly-snot cry at the smallest thing. Even inside, I was thinking, 'This is a bit much, Alex.' I felt broken. I have called it 'Pinocchio disorder' occasionally, as I always used to ask why I 'wasn't a real boy'.

I never felt particularly creative. I studied biology at university because it was the name of one of my subjects at school. I gave it no more thought than that. And at school, I had chosen those subjects because my brothers had chosen the same ones. I had never asked myself what I was actually interested in. I didn't know, as I never had a special interest that lasted for long. I obtained a good degree by persuading my brain that understanding the subject from lecture to lecture was emotionally rewarding, because I would look clever in front of everyone. I was awarded a PhD because I so desperately wanted to be 'Doctor Conner' that I forced it through.

This cost me a lot. By the time I was twenty-six, I was married with a baby. I was a successful professional scientist, people unironically called me 'The Golden Child', and I quite seriously considered suicide.

None of it was real. I was waiting to be a *real boy.*

One of the main ways in which I coped with how I was feeling was by drinking. Alcohol was a significant part of my life from the age of around fourteen or fifteen until my last-ever drink in late 2022. Something I am proud of now is when people tell me that my story of breaking free from my disordered drinking – for reasons of domestic anxiety at 5 p.m. (or whatever time yours is) – helped them to access support to quit. It doesn't matter what we quit (I was also partial to other highs).

Quitting an addiction that is due to ADHD is hard, and it appears to me to be a bit different to other types of addiction. If I have helped one person access support to quit, it will all be worth it. Unless I have inspired more to start drinking with my jokes. Admittedly that would be worse.

Throughout my life, I have been diagnosed and misdiagnosed, ridiculed for thinking something was wrong with me and then praised for my mask. I knew these descriptions of me were wrong, I just didn't know what the right explanation was.

Now I have a small profile as someone interested in ADHD, it feels as if I have suddenly found some ways to describe my brain that make me feel better about myself. I have been labelled my whole life as 'lazy' and 'flippant' and have been told I have a lot of potential (if I only applied myself). I have been told that I have a substance use problem (I do), and that I don't have a substance use problem (I still do). I have been told that I should be myself – yet when I unmask, I am told that I am leaning into 'this ADHD thing' so the mask goes back on. Doctors have called me 'bipolar', 'depressed', 'anxious' and 'neurotic'.

PROLOGUE

But the very worst labels, the most hurtful and damaging ones, are those I have given myself. There is a big difference between intellectually accepting we have ADHD and the longer, slower process of emotionally accepting it. The aim is the latter. I do this by choosing the label of ADHD. I choose it because it means I can start to let go of the painful parts in some way. It means I can plan my future with my ADHD – and this opens up a lot of possibilities.

In response to the frequently asked, 'Why do you need to label?', I reiterate that we already have so many labels from every direction. My view is that labels that restrict our universe should be rejected, while labels that expand our options can be healthy. But most importantly, we get to choose our own label.

ADHD isn't helped by the expectations and constraints of our society, but ADHD isn't a consequence of society either. It is a disorder that restricts my performance, despite my ability, talent, privilege and plans. With the right support and treatment, most of these restrictions are lessened to a point where I find myself at ease with my brain.

A kind of peaceful wildness.

A note from both of us

We met each other pre-diagnosis. James had recently met our co-host and charity powerhouse Sam (James's wife, aka Mrs AuDHD), and Alex had started dating a German law student he met while studying ADHD (not realising that

ADHD UNPACKED

he himself had ADHD for hilarious self-awareness reasons). We got on very well – mainly through insults.

Alex had recently moved to Warwick to take up a job as assistant professor at their medical school and was interviewing for a new scientist to join the team. One of those interviewees was James. He was offered the job and we have worked together ever since. We also shared a broadly negligent approach to work-life that (it turns out) was literally diagnosable. We were excellent at doing some of the work tasks, but we were so easily distracted that we published about ten papers together with very little obvious connection between them.

When James realised he needed to get a handle on the likely fact that he had ADHD and Alex could share a bit of that experience, James started advocating immediately for more awareness and support. Alex claims that watching James do this was a huge inspiration to 'come out' with ADHD, so we started sharing our experiences more widely, combining it with our professional ability to explain the science of ADHD to a wider audience.

We read, heard and watched many things that didn't reflect our reality of living with ADHD, such as the idea that it gets easier with age, or that we are all incredibly creative, or the evidence from the scientific papers we were reading. We wanted a resource that was balanced, aimed at adults with ADHD and broadly accurate. So, we made one.

At some point, James (and we know it was James because we checked our texts) suggested recording our

PROLOGUE

conversations on ADHD as a podcast because we laughed a lot but learnt quite a bit as well. Before long, The ADHD Adults was born. Alex was supposed to register the website name 'Adult ADHD UK', but lost concentration and registered ADHDadultUK by accident. We also brought Sam in – partly because she does all the work for the charity, partly to add some intersectionality to a podcast hosted by two middle-aged white men, and partly because we want our listeners to see that there is always someone out there with worse ADHD symptoms than you. We checked – we're allowed to say that!

Since then, The ADHD Adults podcast has had more than five million listens, we give talks on ADHD all over the world and we have built the charity ADHDadultUK into a support hub for adults who have (or think they have) ADHD and need evidence-based guidance. We are also a growing community of people unkindly but accurately referred to as a 'chaotic squirrel rave'.

We have been supported by a huge number of people, and we hope that our book will give you even more ammunition to get out there and advocate for our community.

CHAPTER 1

What is ADHD?

If you have bought this book, it might worry you that we don't really know the answer to this question. The thing is, there are lots of answers. For many people, 'probably not what you think it is' is an accurate but admittedly not very helpful place to start.

What we do know is that a lot of people are unaware that ADHD even *exists* in adults.[1] Out of those who do, some still believe myths and misconceptions about ADHD, such as the belief that 'ADHD is just a disorder of naughty young boys', for example. For anyone reading this who isn't naughty, or young, or a boy for that matter, we will spend some time on these myths in Chapter 4.

The way in which ADHD symptoms manifest themselves is (currently) thought to be split into two types: inattention and hyperactivity/impulsiveness. There are around nine symptoms of inattentiveness and nine symptoms of hyper-activity/impulsiveness used in the diagnosis. Other lists of symptoms are available, but most people use the ones taken from a book called *The Diagnostic and Statistical*

Manual of Mental Disorders (also known as DSM),[2] which is used by most healthcare professionals in the US and across the world (more on that in Chapter 6). This means it is possible to be diagnosed with one of three 'flavours' of ADHD. You could be diagnosed with inattentive type ADHD only (this used to be called ADD and is also sometimes called inattentive presentation). Or you could (not very commonly) be diagnosed with hyperactive/impulsive type (or presentation) ADHD only. The third and the most common form is the 'full monty' of both types, called combined type ADHD. You will find loads more on all the different types of ADHD and how people get diagnosed in Chapter 6.

If you are one of those people who read prologues, you will know that both of us have combined type ADHD. We are in good company because around a half of adults with ADHD (and probably more) have this form of the disorder (or condition or difference — you of course get to choose which word best describes your own ADHD).

Over history, ADHD has had many names. In 1902, an English paediatrician called Sir George Frederic Still somewhat judgementally referred to what we now call ADHD as an 'abnormal defect of moral control in children',[3] which might be where some of the stigma around ADHD started. Until the 1960s, pretty much all the focus (excuse the terrible pun) on what is now called ADHD was centred on hyperactivity, and in 1968 they added 'hyperkinetic reaction in childhood' to the diagnostic textbook.

It wasn't until 1987 that the name 'attention deficit hyperactivity disorder', or ADHD, was officially recognised. Despite

WHAT IS ADHD?

it being a bit awful and often unhelpful, that name seems to have stuck. Quite incredibly, ADHD in adults wasn't a formal medical diagnosis until 2008, even though it has probably been with us throughout our evolution. It can take a while for the doctors to catch up with the changes. Alex was diagnosed in the UK as recently as 2015, but they still wrote 'hyperkinetic disorder' on the official document instead of ADHD.

Wait, what were we talking about? Oh yeah, ADHD is a really shit name. In fact, attention deficit hyperactivity disorder is, if we are honest, one of the worst names of any medical condition, and this includes the terribly named 'alien hand syndrome' or the fantastic 'coxsackievirus'. (Other real disease names that we discussed for this bit and spent a lot of time hyperfocusing on include 'maple syrup urine disease' and 'slapped cheek syndrome'. We get easily distracted.)

There are several reasons why the name 'attention deficit hyperactivity disorder' is less than helpful. Firstly, there is a pretty clear disconnect between what the medical world thinks a word means and what most of us would usually think it meant. To be fair to scientists and (to a lesser extent) doctors, 'deficit' in medical terms can technically also mean 'impairment'. However, most normal people would interpret 'deficit' as a lack of something or 'less'. So, when people hear that ADHD is an attention deficit, they naturally might assume that people with ADHD have less attention than people without ADHD. This simply isn't true, and it was never meant to be true when they first called it a deficit. It wasn't helpful.

Rather than having *reduced amounts* of attention, most people with ADHD have problems with *allocating* their attention to the right task. All people have limited attention. We would go quite mad if we focused on every bit of information that comes our way, so of course our attention has to be directed towards specific tasks (a task here being any activity or even thought process that enables us to function or thrive). Imagine if we couldn't ever stop paying attention – we would be distracted by every dog barking and every ice cream van in the neighbourhood (these might be bad examples though, because we are distracted by those two things).

Humans do have some level of control over what they choose to pay attention to (but not always). For people with ADHD, we are often less able to 'choose' not only what we pay attention to, but also for how long. This is often not a conscious decision we get to make; rather, the brain does it for us (even if we have planned to do something else).

ADHD can also mean that if we are engaged with something, we can have issues in switching attention from one task to another. This also doesn't always lead to less attention; in fact, at times we can have *way* more attention than usual. Too much even. This is called 'hyperfocus', and we will talk even more about this later (assuming we don't forget).

The name 'attention deficit' seems to play into the hands of those annoying and persistent ADHD myths that we always have less attention in general. This misunderstanding isn't just a bit annoying – it can be a massive barrier for someone with ADHD to seek help in the first place. So many people in our ADHD community have told us that they thought their

WHAT IS ADHD?

periods of hyperfocus excluded them from an ADHD diagnosis, when in fact it would have helped to confirm it.

Let's look at the second part of the name: the hyperactivity part. Again, the name is unhelpful. Firstly, around one third of adults have no major issues with hyperactivity or its connected issue, impulsiveness. This is why you will sometimes hear ADHD referred to as ADD, or attention deficit disorder, particularly in the US. There are also a few research papers suggesting that we split hyperactivity and impulsivity to make it a 'three-dimensional structure' instead of the current 'two-dimensional structure' of ADHD symptoms (we don't know what that would do to the name – ADHID?).

The confusion doesn't stop there. For those of us adults who DO have issues with hyperactivity and/or impulsiveness, these symptoms are often internalised. This can mean that many people with ADHD don't necessarily present themselves as 'fidgety' (as it slightly rudely describes us in the DSM book) or struggling to sit still, which are criteria in the diagnostic manual. Alex always says his brain feels like it is filled with bees, as a description of internalised hyperactivity. For example, if you are the type of person who just can't sunbathe for more than five minutes before getting up and doing something, or find that you can't relax on the sofa in the evening, you may have 'internal restlessness' or feel as if you are 'driven by a motor'. That is just one anecdotal example, of course. Some people with ADHD *love* sunbathing. It also doesn't mean you necessarily have ADHD if you *hate* sunbathing. This is one of the problems with diagnosing disorders that are extreme versions of everyday life: it is very hard to find that line between personality and condition.

The impulsive element of 'hyperactivity/impulsiveness' can include the burning shame of 'not being able to wait your turn in a conversation' or 'interrupting people' all the time. Or even really wanting to, but having to restrain yourself physically or mentally. These things are part of the condition, but as they're not 'hyperactivity', they're not really represented anywhere in the ADHD name.

This idea of having an extremely powerful urge to interrupt and constantly restraining yourself is also not included in the diagnostic manual – and we really think it should be. It can be another cause of missing ADHD (especially in women) as there appears to be a stronger cultural pressure to self-restrict externalised hyperactivity and impulsiveness. We are not just pointing out the gender inequality to look good in front of our lefty friends. It also happens to be true.

There has been a lot of talk about a better name for ADHD but, as of yet, there is no general consensus. We suggest 'intention and emotion regulation disorder', although the word 'disorder' is contentious because ADHD is somewhere between a disorder, a condition and a disability (something we will talk more about later). We also considered 'widespread emotion and intention regulation disorder' but that spells WEIRD and might send the wrong message. More seriously, we would prefer a name that reflects challenges with the intention to do things and the emotions of ADHD. This might work best because many people don't understand that nobody wants to be able to do those things more than us. Our brains just don't let us. It isn't about willpower.

WHAT IS ADHD?

You might have noticed that the name ADHD doesn't include the word 'emotion' anywhere at all (which is why our suggested name does). Why do we care, you might ask? We care because this doesn't make sense. Not everybody with ADHD has issues with all three elements of hyperactivity, impulsivity or inattentiveness. But despite not being central to the diagnostic criteria (yet), pretty much *everybody* with ADHD has issues with regulating their emotional responses. This is called 'emotional dysregulation' and we cover this a lot more in Chapter 11, as it is an important part of ADHD and how to live peacefully with your neurodivergent brain.

So, ADHD can essentially be reduced to challenges with regulating three simple things: attention, emotion and inhibition. Emotional regulation, as we have just discussed, is pretty much a universal problem for people with ADHD. Problems regulating 'attention' is in the title of the disorder, so that is covered (although it isn't *less* attention, remember). The last one – 'inhibition' – refers to our lack of ability to stop ourselves doing or thinking about things (so inhibiting both thoughts and actions). This lack of inhibition means our behaviour can be both impulsive and hyperactive (which is why these are kept together in the diagnosis).

There are lots of examples. We might impulsively buy something on the spur of the moment (it isn't called an impulse purchase by accident) or even engage in 'risky sexual behaviour' (which sounds like an amazing 1980s band name) because we find both of those things rewarding in the heat of the moment. We will explore the concept of reward in more detail in Chapter 10 as this is a bit complex and quite fundamental to understanding a lot of our ADHD behaviours.

What all of this means practically is that we often struggle to inhibit both our mental and physical reactions to events that we know are coming (or even think might be coming). This is called proactive inhibition. And we can struggle in the present with how we inhibit our responses to events as they happen in real time (reactive inhibition). This is why impulsiveness is included with the 'hyperactivity' part of the name ADHD. These are both problems regulating our thoughts and physical reactions.

You may also have noticed that in a chapter on what ADHD is, we have discussed what is wrong with the name and have spent a suspicious amount of time discussing what it isn't. So, what is it?

From a brain science perspective, ADHD is a neurological condition that we are born with. The brain both looks different and acts differently compared to an average person. ADHD can affect many aspects of how someone processes information in their brain and how they act on that information. We tend to share a lot of the same processing challenges, but how that looks (in terms of our symptoms and general behaviour) can be very different, depending on loads of factors: cultural, biological and environmental. For example, somebody might demonstrate their symptoms of impulsiveness through gambling behaviour, whereas a second person might find restricting their impulse shopping more of a behavioural challenge. You might do both, of course.

WHAT IS ADHD?

ADHD is also highly genetic. Although some aspects of ADHD are actually very treatable, it is considered 'incurable' in that it can't be fully treated and never truly goes away. So, ADHD is fundamentally a lifelong neurodevelopmental disorder. This phrase can be really useful if you feel forced to explain your ADHD challenges in a setting in which you aren't feeling safe enough to talk about ADHD more clearly (such as with a shitty boss). Another useful description is 'I have a neurological disorder', which is both accurate and a bit scary for that unpleasant boss in their natural environment of not wanting to get told off.

Let's break that first description down briefly. Lifelong means you are usually born with it, you will have shown signs from early childhood and sadly it isn't going anywhere. As we have said, there is currently no cure for ADHD (although there are some effective treatments for certain aspects, which will be discussed a lot more in Chapter 7).

Straightaway, this idea that ADHD is lifelong has been long accepted by the science but still causes a lot of confusion by ... erm ... also the science. Because how do we deal with the idea that according to much of the medical information we read, not EVERYONE with childhood ADHD goes on to have adult ADHD, yet it is a lifelong incurable disorder? We are no mathematicians, but something isn't adding up here.

In fact, it is far more likely that EVERYONE who has ADHD as a child will grow up to still have ADHD (or at least be neurodivergent). Those adults are therefore either hiding (often called masking) their struggles from the world or at the very least, they are among the lucky ones to have developed a neurodivergent personality of ADHD traits that isn't necessarily a problem in their lives (although that is rare without treatment or support). This throws up another complex talking point for later – that a 'diagnosis' of ADHD might be medical and biological but also includes a subjective social element based on how damaging it is to the person specifically.

The word 'neurodevelopmental' refers to the fact that people with ADHD have brains that develop significantly differently (and slightly more slowly) than average, when compared to the general population. We have to be careful not to say 'compared to normal people' because even though we don't always feel like it, we are still normal in the same way that particularly tall people are still normal people. Choosing the right word isn't always easy but words matter, and the word 'disorder' can also split opinions. Some people don't like to be labelled with a disorder at all and prefer the term 'condition', or in some cases, simply 'difference'.

In medical textbooks (and in the diagnostic criteria), the second 'D' of ADHD stands for disorder because it has a persistent, severe and negative effect on the person in more than one area of their life. Essentially, then, ADHD is the diagnosis of a medical disorder in which our behaviours are affected by the fact that our brains appear to be different to the general population in quite a few areas, both in terms of what those brains look like (neuroanatomy) and how they work (neurophysiology). We will use the word 'disorder' throughout this book, but would never label someone else with a disorder who didn't feel that was appropriate for them.

The stats

ADHD is very common: at least five times as common as type 1 diabetes.[4] Studies have estimated that around 1.9 per cent of adults would meet the criteria for an ADHD diagnosis.[5] Some estimates are even higher, with some studies suggesting that as many as 4.9 per cent of adults have ADHD.[6] Even the lower figure of 1.9 per cent is a lot of people.

People you know, people you love, people you are related to, people you walk past in the street ... Around one in forty of them have ADHD. Of those people though, most of them either don't know ADHD exists in adults, don't think (or don't know) they have it, or are waiting to be assessed by a professional. These 'undiagnosed' ADHD adults probably make up around 80 to 90 per cent of people with ADHD (according to our figures based on NHS ADHD medication prescription data – that was a fun afternoon of sums). This is a huge group of people who are likely to have spent their whole lives just thinking they are a bit rubbish and wondering why they can't do the simple things that others seem to find so easy. We both spent decades thinking exactly that.

What do these people have in common? Well, even though we are all kind of different (this is one of the problems faced by doctors in diagnosing ADHD properly), we can start to spot some of the behaviours and symptoms you might be likely to see. It is important to keep in mind that not all of these will be seen in everyone with ADHD, of course. Having said that, one common observation is that we are more likely to be naturally disorganised (a lot more than most people). We might be (or feel) restless, or we might lack the motivation to do anything at all. We also might appear to the outside world to be massively organised, having learnt that extreme control is the only way to survive a natural lack of organisational skills.

This 'masking' can come at an enormous personal and emotional cost and, depending on how it fits your individual personality, can be very unhealthy. This is why it is difficult to diagnose ADHD without a mental health professional. Of course, most organised people aren't hiding ADHD, and many people with ADHD have found healthy ways to stay more organised. This is why assessment and communication are so important, as the behaviours can appear very different, even for the same symptoms. It is the cost to the person (emotionally and physically) and the effect on those around them that has to be assessed.

Adults with ADHD may also be overtly emotional or appear forgetful. Some might be very withdrawn, whereas others appear highly energetic or extroverted. How we respond to living with ADHD can vary from person to person and change over our lifetime. But equally, many of us might appear absolutely 'typical' to most independent observers. This is because many people with ADHD learn to hide or 'mask' their symptoms to try to fit in. We wear these masks because our traits and behaviours are generally not particularly well received in society.

Have you ever seen an advert for a job that says 'Seeking someone who will struggle to turn up on time, may forget their laptop, will only intermittently be able to finish tasks and will sit and daydream in longer meetings'? We are guessing not. We often hide our true selves, such as being constantly anxious about timekeeping rather than always being late, sometimes to the point where we can appear from the outside to get through life reasonably well (on the surface), until life events such as going to university or going through the menopause cause our coping strategies to unravel, and our symptoms or traits become all too evident.

Masking is a huge part of the lives of many adults with ADHD, especially those seemingly 'high achievers' or those with responsibilities (such as carers). It is a very important and highly misunderstood element of living with ADHD because many people might think that if we can mask our symptoms, then surely we are 'doing' those things we claim to struggle with – isn't that just willpower? We have heard that all our lives and still do (in fact, this is a myth that we will discuss a lot more in Chapter 4).

The main element is that the masking uses a degree of cognitive freedom and an awful lot of energy (James describes this as bandwidth). We can't do it all the time without an enormous emotional and physical toll. It is like telling someone that they managed to run up one flight of stairs, so with willpower they should easily be able to run to the top of the Empire State Building.

The emotional and physical toll of ADHD

We sometimes refer to the cost of living in a neurotypical world as the 'burden' of ADHD. We generally don't mean the burden of us on society (although there is significant financial cost associated with having us undiagnosed and untreated in society). We are more concerned by the burdens on our own mental and physical well-being (and those around us). This next bit isn't particularly funny and often comes as a bit of a shock to people who think ADHD is a sort of funny modern quirk (like a goatee beard). ADHD is the mental health condition that has the most significant negative effects on the largest number of people in the entire world of psychiatric medicine. It isn't a quirk.

Before we get to some of the more sobering statistics, the fantastic news is that with the right support, almost all of those increased 'personal burdens' faced by adults with ADHD can be reduced to the same level as the rest of the population (notice that we can't get rid of them completely). This support includes access to medication for those who want it, but should also include access to non-medical treatments (such as therapy). We also need changes to our school and work structures so we have an environment that encourages reasonable adjustments and different ways of achieving goals. This isn't about special treatment. This is about removing barriers so we can be as successful as anybody else at whatever it is we choose to do (within reason). Our current system means that without diagnosis and support, adults with ADHD face:

- an increased risk of reduced quality of life

- an increased risk of relationship breakdown

- an increased risk of substance use issues, gambling and debt

WHAT IS ADHD?

- increased unemployment or under-employment

- less access to higher education, or staying in it

- an increased risk of criminality (30.2 per cent of prisoners have ADHD symptoms)

- increased accidental injuries

- an increased suicide risk

- an increased risk of premature death

- economic burden for self (the so-called ADHD tax).

The frustrating thing is that the cost of treatment is far lower than NOT supporting adults with ADHD. A Danish study found that it costs the taxpayer an estimated extra 20,000 euros per year in medical bills, lost taxes and other societal costs NOT to diagnose and support an adult with ADHD.[7] With a relatively inexpensive treatment regime, that cost comes down to pretty much zero.

SUMMARY

ADHD is a lifelong neurological condition. If diagnosed and treated (and with the right support), it can become a difference where the challenges we have faced give us new perspectives and enable us to see the world slightly unusually, but not holding us back from the same chance of success as anybody else. Without that support, the consequences can be incredibly severe.

Wherever you are on your ADHD journey, if you have or think you may have ADHD, the signs were probably there early in your childhood, and your ADHD was more than likely to be a gift from the genes of your parents. But what are the causes of ADHD, and do we all get it the same way?

CHAPTER 2

What causes ADHD?

We thought about calling this chapter 'ADHD is your parents' fault', but we weren't 100 per cent sure that people would get the joke about genetics being an important factor rather than bad parenting (and we didn't want a barrage of angry complaints). One of the most common questions about ADHD is 'What causes it?' but the answer might not be what you expect. The most accurate answer right now is 'nobody really knows completely'. We do know some things though, so let's have a look at them.

When trying to understand the causes of ADHD, it is worth comparing it to something very well understood, such as obesity. The causes of obesity are a combination of genetic factors (for example, different people's genes can make different amounts of hunger hormones) and psychological factors (such as stress). There are also a number of additional 'risk factors' for becoming obese that we can look out for. So, obesity is caused by a combination of several things. ADHD is likely to be a similar mix but with genetics being the major factor.

It is important to remember that 'risk factors' are just statistical connections; these are not causes and aren't 100 per cent correct all of the time. People tend to over-interpret a statistical connection and assume one definitely causes the other.[8] But in actual fact, these statistical connections could easily be a total coincidence, such as how organic food sales have increased at the same rate as autism diagnoses over the past fifty years. Of course, organic food isn't a risk factor for having autism, and nor are vaccines or genetically modified foods.[9]

The other common mistake is when two things are linked because of a connected factor, called a confounding variable. A great example of a confounding variable is the joke among statisticians that ice creams are very dangerous, because every year the number of shark attacks increases with the number of ice creams sold. Does that make ice cream a risk factor for shark attacks? Probably not. It is, of course, more likely that both of those factors increase due to sunny weather, putting people in the mood for ice creams and swimming. Sunny weather, therefore, would be the confounding variable!

When we look again at the risk factors for obesity, these are pretty clearly understood. Ironically, these might also be risk factors for ADHD (such as alcohol use and educational level) and almost too ironically, another risk factor for obesity is untreated ADHD. Funding for ADHD research has historically been much lower than for obesity, so concrete evidence for the causes of ADHD is lacking. We don't even know for sure what the 'risk factors' are for ADHD, but the research gives us enough compelling science to suggest which factors are *likely* to be involved.

WHAT CAUSES ADHD?

In this chapter, we will explore some of the likely causes and risk factors, and in Chapter 4, we will smash some common ADHD myths and malingering misinformation about what doesn't cause it (spoiler alert: ADHD is *not* caused by mobile phones or sugary drinks).

What we DO know is that ADHD is a biological, neurodevelopmental disorder that we have from early childhood and probably earlier (as we talked about in Chapter 1). There is currently almost no evidence for an adult-onset form of ADHD, despite so many people (including us) receiving our diagnoses as adults. For most people, those symptoms and traits were always there and, from a medical perspective, must have been there during their childhood in order to get a diagnosis. This may change in the future, but at the moment we don't have enough evidence to support a form of ADHD that can start later in life. Having said that, as many late-diagnosed ADHD adults will tell you, ADHD can get so much more difficult to live with, and people often confuse that with a form of 'adult-onset' ADHD. They often let us know quite angrily on the internet.

The good news is that it is only a matter of time before we can start to fill in these gaps in the science, but we can already start to make some educated conclusions about the causes of ADHD.

ADHD and genetics

What we do know (almost certainly) is that ADHD is largely a genetic disorder, which means the main reason we have it lies in our DNA. Inside almost all of the many trillion living cells of your body sits your genetic material, or DNA. The very same DNA, although a bit changed over time, that you inherited from your biological parents. You inherited about half of it from one (biological) parent, and half from the other.

DNA is quite a boring molecule, unless you are a geneticist when ... No, it is still boring, sorry. It sits there, tightly coiled and ready to leap into action by acting as a blueprint to enable cells to make more useful things, such as proteins.

Insulin is a good example of a protein. People with type 1 diabetes inject themselves with insulin every day because that protein isn't made in their body but is needed to eat bread, sugar and other carbohydrates. Every human has an insulin gene in all of the cells of their body, but every cell doesn't need the insulin protein to be made. So, the gene is only used by a tiny fraction of those cells as a blueprint (much like the blueprint for a building) to make insulin. This needs to be a good blueprint though. Otherwise, when the building is made, the doors might not close properly and the plumbing might not work, but equally there may be a fun slide instead of the stairs. The reason people with type 1 diabetes don't make insulin isn't because the gene is missing, but because the body has killed off the cells (normally found in our pancreas) that are able to read the insulin-gene blueprint and so almost no insulin is made.

So even with genes, there are different reasons why things don't work (and we will see that may be true in ADHD too). Normally, the gene (DNA blueprint) is read by the correct cell (architect) to make the protein (building). This is brilliantly

WHAT CAUSES ADHD?

called 'the central dogma' of biology, and it can go badly wrong if any of those three elements goes wrong.

Only about 1 per cent of your DNA is organised into these blueprints or 'genes'. You have around 50,000 genes in total (not just you – humans in general), but only around 20,000 of those are blueprints for making proteins. Of those 20,000, a whopping third of them are needed to build your brain and keep it working. Therefore, if your DNA isn't quite right, a lot can go wrong and there is a high chance that this could affect your brain.

The other 30,000 genes that aren't a blueprint (or genetic code) for a protein are called non-coding regions. Those non-coding regions are also very important because changes to these areas can be linked to your chances of ADHD development (and pretty much every other aspect of your biology). When we look at your genetic profile as a whole, the 'typical' protein-making genes for brain development might be absolutely fine, but if they aren't regulated properly by DNA differences somewhere else, this could explain why you have ADHD (and many other conditions or differences).

In other words, the building's blueprint (the gene) might be mutated or damaged (like in cystic fibrosis), or the gene might be fine but there could still be a problem with how the blueprint is read (involving other bits of DNA in the same cells). There could also be a problem with the cell itself, like that example of some people with type 1 diabetes where the insulin gene and its regulating DNA might be fine but indirect problems with other genes are destroying the cells that would normally be translating that insulin gene and building

ADHD UNPACKED

a normal working insulin protein – so destroying the architect and the blueprints and the office they work in.[10]

It doesn't stop there. On top of the 20,000 genes that make proteins, and the other 30,000 genes that do … erm … other stuff, there is still even more DNA that collectively makes up your chromosomes and does many other things that scientists have no clue about. OK, maybe a small clue. Sorry, scientists.

In fact, up to 8 per cent of your DNA is actually viral DNA (or it was once), having been inserted into your DNA by viruses over the last few millions of years and sticking around as we evolved. So, you are quite literally part virus (again, not just you – this isn't a series of personal attacks) and as much as 4 per cent of your DNA is Neanderthal. It is probably best not to overthink how we got that 4 per cent of Neanderthal DNA.

Wherever our DNA came from originally, it has changed (mutated) over the years and is still changing and mutating right now. Our job is to ask, from an ADHD perspective, what are the consequences of these changes? What has happened to your DNA blueprint genes, or the other DNA that controls things, and which genes are affected in ADHD traits?

If any of these genes get altered by mistake as a cell divides, or on exposure to radiation (including sunshine) or chemicals (such as those found in cigarette smoke), a genetic mutation can occur. This means that your DNA blueprint may not be read, or too easily read, by your cells, or it may

36

produce a protein that looks and works differently, or not at all. As so many genes are involved in brain development, there is obviously a lot that could go wrong after a mutation.

Fortunately, the VAST majority of those genetic mutations are repaired by our body as they happen (or we would be riddled with cancer all the time). On top of that, most of this happens in cells that we don't use to make babies. These are called somatic cells, and even though they can be harmful for that person, they don't get passed on to the next generation.

From a population perspective, the serious effects happen when one of those 'genetic mutations' occurs in our sperm or egg cells (or the parts of the body that make those cells). These are called germ cells. The sperm are made in the fantastically named 'seminiferous tubules'. If that isn't a forest in the *Lord of the Rings*, then it really should have been. These mutations in germ cells are the ones that can get passed to the next generation. While that feels a bit scary – that mutations can be passed down to our children – it is also the reason for evolution and why we don't all look the same. If we didn't pass on loads of mutations, we would all be single-celled organisms swimming around an endless sea.

The observation that ADHD is genetic began when people started to realise that ADHD traits often run in families. Many studies have looked at the DNA of people with ADHD to try to understand the condition and how we inherit it. The big problem with these observations, of course, is that 'running in families' can also be environmental, as most families share an environment as well as genes. For example, it isn't a genetic predisposition to follow a certain religion, but if you looked at the likelihood of religious affiliation, it might appear that there was a genetic element to this, as someone's religion as an adult also very often appears to 'run in families'.

This is a huge and not fully solved limitation of trying to prove if ADHD runs in families because of our genes or because of that shared environment. It isn't possible to design studies that control for all environmental effects. What we can do is design different studies that at least try to mitigate their effect on the results. When you do this, it tells you what the impact of that 'shared environment' was likely to have been on the chances of ADHD developing. Before we go through those, the main result suggests that growing up with a 'shared environment' doesn't have a major effect; it is the genes themselves that are mostly responsible for ADHD (this shouldn't be controversial but often is).

Some of that research involved comparing the DNA of identical twins (because they are born with almost identical DNA codes). Other studies compared entire distant families (who share some genes but might have grown up very differently and far apart), as well as adopted people and their biological relatives. These are all useful as they help us understand the impact of our genetics compared to that of growing up in a shared environment.

These studies have generally agreed that ADHD is about 70 to 80 per cent genetic.[11] This is a very rough estimate depending on what you mean by genetic and lots of other

WHAT CAUSES ADHD?

things. That is the problem with genetics. It is a bit wobbly. To explain that 70 to 80 per cent figure ... If you take two identical twins who have been adopted from birth and raised in different homes, if one of them has ADHD, the other one has around a 70 to 80 per cent chance of also having ADHD. It is also worth noting that social factors, including access to a diagnosis of ADHD in the first place, will influence this chance.

Another relevant finding from the studies (genetically speaking) is that if a close relative of yours, such as a parent, child or sibling, has ADHD, you are between five and nine times more likely to also have ADHD than a randomly selected member of the general population. Armed with all this knowledge, it is fair to say that ADHD is largely genetic.

But you might ask, if it is genetic then why isn't it 100 per cent? Why don't both identical twins always have ADHD? This is a good and difficult question. Firstly, there are social and psychological reasons. The test for ADHD is affected by lots of factors that can be inconsistent or difficult to standardise. These could be anything from somebody's perspectives on their own traits, how much their symptoms impact them on a day-to-day basis, or even any bias in the opinion or ability of the doctor doing the assessment in the first place. We also don't have a blood test for ADHD (yet), so an accurate diagnosis of borderline cases can be difficult. All of this can reduce that number. To understand more about how ADHD is diagnosed in general, head to Chapter 6.

We also know there is no single 'ADHD gene' causing the condition (and, in fact, any single-gene diseases are very rare in general). Someone with ADHD would often have dozens or even hundreds of small mutations in genes needed for brain development. None of those on their own would have much of a disruptive effect on the brain, but collectively all of those little changes are thought to lay the foundations for our brains developing and working differently. This means that both of your parents could donate half of the 'ADHD genes' without having enough to reach ADHD levels themselves. It is even possible (because we all have two lots of genes, one from each parent) that both of your parents had ADHD but didn't pass on ADHD genes to you. This is statistically very unlikely though.

The last reason why this isn't 100 per cent genetic is that the mutations that tipped you over the edge into ADHD might have happened in your body very early in your development (when you were just a few cells) or in the sperm- or egg-making germ cells of your parents. Then they would NOT necessarily have ADHD, but YOU could have it. You would be the ADHD pioneer of the family. Equally, if you had ADHD-causing genes but you developed mutations in your sperm or eggs that changed them, your children might not develop ADHD.

You may notice we haven't talked about epigenetics here (environmental changes to genes that we can then pass on). This idea is too early in its infancy to make meaningful conclusions for ADHD. There isn't enough evidence to support epigenetics and ADHD yet (but it is interesting).

It is clear that genes play a big part in the development of ADHD, but that isn't the full story. We know that there are

WHAT CAUSES ADHD?

many people who believe that ADHD is purely a result of emotional trauma and/or society being structurally incompatible with adults with ADHD. A number of more populist (and usually self-described) ADHD specialists routinely claim that ADHD is not genetic but is reversible and caused by things that happened during childhood. This isn't correct but it isn't without some elements that are worth exploring. To do this, we have to look at the potential impact of the environment on developing ADHD.

ADHD and the environment

We know that ADHD is rarely entirely down to one thing, and as we've noted, research is very much in its infancy. However, there is NO meaningful evidence that social factors (including emotional trauma) are solely responsible for directly causing ADHD. This statement can often frustrate people.

What we have is evidence that differences in our genes provide some form of 'likelihood bonfire' for ADHD. We don't know if we need a metaphorical match to light that bonfire (such as head trauma) OR if it just lights spontaneously. We also know that people with ADHD have measurable differences in their neurology but those brain differences are not the same for everyone with ADHD — we will explore that in a lot more detail in Chapter 3.

As well as the enormous genetic component, developing ADHD appears to be more complex and different for each person. For some, ADHD is entirely defined by their genetics. This may be something that they were always going to have, wherever, however and whenever they were born and raised. For others, it may be that their ADHD 'genetic bonfire' required a different type of match, so their ADHD lies in a combination of gene differences and an environmental trigger.

Where it gets controversial involves the precise nature of what those environmental triggers are. The sorts of triggers that we currently have strong evidence for are generally things that have a quite measurable, biological effect on our brain. These triggers can include serious head accidents, being exposed to toxic substances (such as cigarette smoke or high levels of alcohol) during our development, or extreme nutritional deprivation early in our lives.

What we don't have is a lot of solid evidence for a form of ADHD occurring solely due to environmental factors (without a genetic predisposition to ADHD in the first place). This is hard to prove, because conditions such as head trauma, epilepsy or post-traumatic stress disorder (PTSD) – and even fundamental elements of the human experience (such as menopause) – can present symptoms in a very similar way to those of ADHD (for similar reasons) and exacerbate the symptoms of people who also have ADHD.

Many researchers have tried to identify (with varying degrees of success) some of the exact environmental factors that are associated with someone developing ADHD. The word 'associated' is important in that last sentence, because environmental factors aren't (usually) thought to cause ADHD on their own, but combine with our genes to facilitate the brain

WHAT CAUSES ADHD?

developing differently. These environmental elements are more likely to be those 'risk factors' we discussed earlier in the chapter. There seems to be a clear, increased risk of developing ADHD after exposure to:

- toxins, including lead and mercury

- environmental pollution

- prenatal (before birth) exposure to alcohol

- exposure to cigarette smoke (in the womb and possible in early childhood)

- low nutritional health as a child.

Annoyingly for us trying to get answers, these studies are often poorly designed or poorly funded smaller trials. This means it is difficult to know if those environmental factors are just associated but not heavily involved in causing ADHD itself.

One environmental factor that appears to trigger ADHD is severe early deprivation. Some of this evidence came from distressing research looking at the increased levels of ADHD in people who were children in Romanian orphanages.[12] These children faced horribly deprived, neglected and extremely traumatic conditions. We don't know which elements of that environment were the exact trigger, or even if there was just one.[13]

There is also research showing that some things are clearly *not* factors responsible for ADHD. This includes exposure to computers, parenting style (outside of severe deprivation, of course), video games, educational quality or having friends with ADHD. What the evidence *does* show is that ADHD is a neurological disorder that is highly genetic. Compare ADHD to any other neurological condition (anxiety, depression, etc.) and you start to realise that ADHD is probably the single most genetically determined psychological disorder/condition.

The sheer level of variability from person to person, and the complexity of ADHD, is very often and widely misunderstood. Both medical professionals and researchers still don't know a lot about many aspects of ADHD. Science is often filled with these unknowns, especially with mental health conditions. Unfortunately, this creates a knowledge vacuum that can be quickly filled with less evidence-based ideas, well-meaning (but completely wrong) 'common sense' and downright amoral quackery. It is important that we have a clear sense of why these myths and misunderstandings are wrong. We will talk about this a lot more in Chapter 4 and discuss how to compassionately communicate the real evidence to others. At the very least, it might help you feel a bit smug!

Trauma and ADHD

It is very common for us to be told that our ADHD is caused by early-childhood trauma. There are many reasons why people might believe this, largely due to popular books that promote this theory. When you look at the evidence, it becomes clear why this is a controversial area.

WHAT CAUSES ADHD?

Psychological trauma could be considered to be an 'environmental trigger', alongside the other triggers we have mentioned earlier, including physical trauma, such as traumatic brain injury (which accounts for fewer than 15 per cent of people with ADHD). It is important to separate these two types of trauma, as the respective evidence for their roles in ADHD is very different.

The first issue with psychological trauma being a trigger for the development of ADHD is that, in most cases, environmental triggers occur in the perinatal period (just before and after birth). Most childhood traumas take place long after this time. The second issue becomes clear when you look at the long-lasting symptoms of psychological trauma: fidgeting, inattentiveness, hyperactivity and impulsivity, issues with organisation, emotional dysregulation, and others. You can be excused if you think the last sentence got missed in editing, as it clearly looks like a list of ADHD symptoms. And there is the rub: trauma can cause lifelong, ADHD-like symptoms without actually causing ADHD. There is a significant crossover between the symptoms of both, and therefore misdiagnosis can happen.

Looking at scientific studies, there is evidence of a link between psychological trauma and ADHD, but it is a link that goes both ways. So, for example, if you have ADHD, you are more likely to have post-traumatic stress disorder (PTSD), and if you have PTSD, you are more likely to have ADHD. But this is a correlation, and it doesn't tell you which causes which, or if another confounding variable is causing both.

Biologically, childhood trauma can cause changes in brain development, but these are generally different changes to those seen in ADHD. These changes can, however, lead to the ADHD-like symptoms listed earlier, and these can, if untreated, last a lifetime. It is easy to understand how people can see a link between the two, especially after reading popular books stating that ADHD is a response to psychological trauma and then making the leap to 'ADHD is caused by trauma'. This isn't what the evidence says, and it invalidates the experience of most people with ADHD. We also tend not to 'repress' bad memories. In fact, we have evolved memories partly to remember bad things so we can avoid them in the future.

Importantly, as ADHD is a neurodevelopmental condition, a trauma that occurs later in life is unlikely to cause ADHD. Essentially, early life psychological trauma can and probably does contribute to the risk of developing ADHD in some people, but in relatively few cases compared to other environmental triggers.

WHAT CAUSES ADHD?

SUMMARY

ADHD is almost always caused by some combination of genetic and/or environmental factors. For most adults with ADHD, this comes from inherited genetic mutations. But for a significant other group, this may have been due to new, spontaneous mutations or even triggered (or caused) by an early life environmental factor that causes the brain to develop differently.[14]

Although (usually physical) trauma can be an ADHD trigger, it is also highly probable that people who already have ADHD will have subsequently faced more adversity growing up than average. So it should be considered that they may have faced relatively higher levels of trauma mainly because of living with ADHD.

This is why working with adults with ADHD should be approached in a trauma-informed manner – this means we should always assume that traumatic events may be playing a role in the person's life. We tend to split our discussion of trauma and ADHD into the physical serious traumatic events (such as deprivation and car accidents), serious emotional trauma, and other perspectives that felt traumatic despite the apparent feeling in a neurotypical society that these might not appear traumatic to most people.

We also try not to refer to non-neurodivergent people as 'neurotypical' because we find it can be unhelpful to label people from groups we don't belong to – and especially because the concept of neurotypical isn't a formal scientific term and doesn't necessarily refer to any one individual but to a hypothetical, statistical average of every mental trait. We also certainly don't condone the alternative term, 'muggles', despite how funny that may be to say.

Whatever the true cause of ADHD, the one definite truth is that this is a difference in how the brain works, what it looks like and how it communicates with itself and the rest of the body. In the next chapter, we will look at those brain differences and see how they can help explain much of the elements of ADHD in adults.

CHAPTER 3

ADHD and the brain

If ADHD is caused by the brain developing differently, it is probably helpful to start by brainsplaining (we have definitely not made this word up). The human brain is an incredible thing. Every thought, feeling, memory, sensation, plan and emotion you have ever felt happened right there, in that floppy mass of fatty tissue inside your skull.

Your brain contains around 100 billion neurons.[15] This figure might be coming down slightly in the more recent estimates to about 80 billion, but nobody really knows the exact number because ... how would you count them? There are a lot of neurons anyway, and these are connected to the rest of your body (often through your spinal column) to enable information to come in and go out again.

As the brain is so complex, there are many ways of separating it into specific areas, and these areas have different roles. Some brain areas are easy to identify as they look different to the areas around them, but many others aren't easily separated into fixed parts with specific

ADHD UNPACKED

roles. It would be a bit like trying to identify which part of a Dalmatian dog was the spotty bit.

It might be helpful to first cover the three big parts of the brain. Brain areas often have ridiculously over-complicated anatomical names. Throughout this book, we will try to avoid using them. If we do mention some of the weirder-sounding brain areas (such as the indusium griseum, which sounds like a Harry Potter spell), we will try to break the names down to make them marginally less confusing.

The most primitive and ancient part of the brain, known as the hindbrain, sits deep down towards the back of the head. This brain area, which is very similar in many other animals, coordinates a lot of our vital functions such as breathing and heart rate. Some people refer to it as our 'lizard brain', which is one of those combinations of sort of helpful and wildly wrong that crop up all the time in popular science slang. This part of the brain is ancient because it formed first, but it has also been evolving for this whole time as well.

Travelling outwards, next comes the midbrain – along with hindbrain and forebrain, these are anatomy words even we can handle. They literally mean the back bit, middle bit and front-y bit. The midbrain largely acts as a connection between the hindbrain and the last section, the forebrain (closest to the forehead).

The forebrain is the largest part of the human brain and easily the most interesting part in terms of ADHD. This is where important brain functions, such as thinking, planning, organising, language processing, sensory processing

ADHD AND THE BRAIN

and movement, are controlled. You may notice that many of those forebrain functions (apart from movement) are things that humans do pretty well, but most of the other creatures on the planet are less well suited for them (such as organising a party or controlling emotions in an argument). These are sometimes called 'higher functions'. We think this is a bit arrogant considering that some 'lesser' animals can fly up to 11,000 feet high or run at 130 km per hour, while we are hairless apes who often trip over while putting our socks on!

You have probably heard of the 'pre-frontal cortex' part of the forebrain where a lot of this planning happens. Those plans have to be sent to all other parts of the brain, and this communication seems to be disrupted in most people with ADHD (actually, probably all of them).

A lot of research has discovered how these three brain areas (mostly made up of brain cells called neurons) manage to coordinate all of the incredible activities that you do every day. The answer is that they pass messages to each other, like children sending each other notes in class. These notes are in the form of tiny chemical messages called neurotransmitters. A neurotransmitter is hundreds of times smaller than even a single cell in the human body, moving between neurons pretty much all the time. A single bacterium is about one hundred times smaller than a human cell, and these neurotransmitter messages are so small that you could fit tens of millions of them into a single bacterial cell.

Neurotransmitters pass from one neuron of the brain to other neurons (or to another part of the body) across a very small gap measuring just 0.00000002 metres wide (also called 20 nanometres or 20 nm). Before we publish this book, one of us really has to check that number. It is hard with ADHD to count all those zeroes! Hopefully, none of our readers will check if we forgot any.

When the neurotransmitters cross this gap (which is called a synapse), they bind to a specific 'receptor' on the next neuron in the chain (like a key fitting into a lock). Once the receptor has been triggered, this activates the new neuron in the chain. This enables neurons to communicate rapidly – it takes less than one thousandth of a second for a signal to pass from one neuron to the next. Or if it has reached the last neuron in the chain, the neurotransmitter message talks to your arm or leg or whatever. That is some complex biology right there.

Finally, to stop the brain being overactive, the neurotransmitters are then removed from the synapse through a hole that takes them back into the original neuron. Imagine that a child passing notes in a classroom is holding up a message that says 'dance' (for example), so the other children are dancing. The child would then have to take that sign away so that the other children know they should now stop dancing. For the brain to stop us from doing something (such as dancing), the message also has to be taken away.

In the brain, the messages (those neurotransmitters) drain away from the gap (the synaptic cleft) back into the first neuron from where they came originally. Think of it like water draining from the bath when you pull the plug out. This is probably not a perfect analogy, but it is one that will

ADHD AND THE BRAIN

be useful later on when we talk about how the ADHD medications work.

Much like some of James's tips for living with ADHD, the individual parts of the brain on their own are a bit useless. In order to actually get things done, the brain forms a colossal number of interconnected networks. By colossal, we mean around 100 trillion neuron connections talking to each other all the time (a trillion is a million million. Unimaginably large). This is like having a tiny internet inside your skull, with computers in London being permanently connected and talking to computers in Berlin, New Orleans and Brisbane all the time, not just when you send an email.

These neurons can all connect (and talk) to many other neurons at the same time, which in turn connect to other neurons to form networks in the brain. The brain networks are essential for complex brain functions, such as language, emotion and attention, and, just like the internet, they need a solid connection to do this.

Now you may be thinking, 'If I wanted a biology lesson, I'd go and study biology.' You will be glad to know that we are done explaining how neurons and networks form, but ALL of this will make sense later on. Probably.

Why are these networks so important and different in ADHD?

If you were paying attention earlier (pun very much intended), you might remember that we said ADHD is a neurodevelopmental disorder. This is one of quite a few disorders in which the brain hasn't developed in a 'typical' fashion, which causes some impairments in how the brain thinks and does things. Some parts of the brains of people with ADHD (including us) developed differently compared to the brains of people without ADHD. This difference seems to be both in the way the brain looks and in the way it works.

There are several types of brain networks, but going into them in detail would probably make you put this book down and never read it again. Quite a few of these networks are thought to not work properly in at least some of the brains of people with ADHD (or they work in a different way compared to everybody else). The first of these is, wait for it, the cortico-striato-thalamo-cortical loop, or the CSTC loop as it is better known (you might want to say the name slowly or never think about it again). As the name suggests, this brain circuit is a loop, going back to where it starts from. Within this loop are several other individual networks that regulate sustained attention, emotions, selective attention, hyperactivity and an impulsivity circuit. This 'loop' regulates pretty much all the stuff that collectively makes up ADHD. And in ADHD, it works fine. Only joking – it really doesn't.

This might be a good time to say that the research is usually done on averaging the brain studies from many people. At the individual level, each one of those brain networks could work fine in someone with ADHD. We don't all have problems with every network that could be disrupted. That is why the symptoms are different for all of us, and why it is

ADHD AND THE BRAIN

difficult to diagnose. It would be great if we could just look at a single brain network and say 'Yes, that's ADHD', but we can't do this yet.

In addition to the CSTC loop, we have the default mode network or DMN, which is associated with thoughts about ourselves and mind-wandering (we often call this the DeMoN network, because it causes us to daydream when we shouldn't, like the devil ... might). Mind-wandering is covered in Chapter 8, but the name kind of gives it away. Usually, in non-ADHD people (which is as close as we get to saying 'neurotypical people'), this daydreaming network gets switched off when we start a task, by yet another brain group called the 'task-positive network' (or TPN). But that switch appears to be a bit broken in ADHD and the demonic DMN stays on even when the TPN is activated. This is one of the many reasons we can be inattentive: our mind can wander during a task at the drop of a hat.

Among several other brain networks that don't fully operate in ADHD is the 'fronto-parietal' network or 'front-y bit joined to the upper bit at the back' network (but in Latin). This network helps to control attention and executive functions. If you are really trying to read these complex brain anatomy names but struggle to pay attention, you could blame that part of your brain.

It might seem relatively obvious now, but it took a viral epidemic that affected the brains of children in the early twentieth century, causing ADHD-like symptoms, to point doctors at the time towards ADHD being brain-related.[16]

This viral encephalitis lethargica epidemic spread around the world between around 1917 and 1928 and affected approximately 20 million people, often being fatal. Doctors also started to notice 'strange behaviours' in some children who survived it. This included personality changes, emotional instability, learning difficulties, sleep issues, physical tics, depression and poor coordination.

It has since become well established (by medical scientists, possibly not by the media) that brain changes and ADHD go hand in hand. Despite this, and despite what many online videos appear to claim, there is no such thing as a single 'ADHD brain'. Obviously, people sometimes use the term 'ADHD brain' as a short way of saying 'some of the things we tend to have in common'. In fact, we are fairly certain that we have probably said it ourselves on occasion.

Even within our community of people with ADHD, our brains are all gloriously (and annoyingly) different, which is why there isn't a simple brain scan to enable a doctor to say, 'Congratulations, you have ADHD!' (although maybe 'congratulations' isn't the right word, but you know what we mean). This is similar to the fact that the average man is taller than the average woman; nobody realistically thinks that every single man is taller than every single woman or that if you heard someone was five foot six inches, it would automatically mean they were female. (If you prefer metres to feet, five foot six is about 167.64 cm − it is strange that the metric system for height isn't more popular.) The same is true of the differences in the brains of adults with ADHD. Despite that variability, we

ADHD AND THE BRAIN

can start to spot certain brain elements that look different (on average), and these are really useful to help us understand some of the reasons why people with ADHD might do the things they do.

What we know from brain scan studies is that as well as 'network issues', some specific parts of the brain work differently with ADHD. Examples include the 'reward centre' (covered in Chapter 10), the amygdala, which means 'almond' because of its shape and regulates processing of emotions (covered in Chapter 11), the anterior cingulate cortex (which means front bit of the thing that looks like a belt on the outside bit of the brain) and the posterior cingulate cortex (which means the back bit of that same belt structure), which helps to filter out internal and external distractions so we can pay attention to things (covered in Chapter 8). ADHD is also more likely to be different in the basal ganglia, which is involved in movement and hyperactivity (covered in Chapter 9) but we don't know what 'ganglion' means. It seems to be something Latiny-Greek made up by Hippocrates, who also made up that medical oath thing.

SUMMARY

ADHD is a developmental difference in the human brain, which is an incredibly complex organ that regulates all the emotions, behaviours and decisions we make, as well as controlling what goes on in our body. There is a lot of evidence that in ADHD specifically, the areas of the brain that regulate attention, emotions and thinking skills, such as organisation, planning and inhibiting ourselves, look and work just slightly differently than they do (on average) in the general population. These differences in the brain are largely the reason why people with ADHD have their challenges.

This information about brain differences should be enough to persuade people that ADHD is a real, measurable neurological disorder. It is a biological phenomenon that can be treated to a certain degree with drugs that change the amounts of those neurotransmitters (called neuromodulators). We can see differences in the average brains and predict the likely ADHD profile of the children of people with ADHD (if not yet predict a specific diagnosis). Unfortunately, all that evidence doesn't account for the inability of many people to actually read evidence and allow it to inform their opinion (we really need to teach this in schools). The degree to which pervasive, damaging and blatantly false explanations, rumours and myths gain traction in the world of ADHD is nothing short of staggering.

In the next chapter, we are going to have a look at a few of the more powerful myths and misunderstandings of what ADHD is. We will also explore how it affects people and hopefully arm you with the facts so you can argue back when faced with accusations and stigma-inducing nonsense. You don't have to argue back or even reply to those people though. It is often more than enough to be smug in the knowledge that you know more than they do!

CHAPTER 4

Myth-understandings!

It is hard not to notice quite a few persistent and completely incorrect myths surrounding ADHD, which seem to be quite prevalent in the media and more broadly accepted in society. These myths collectively add to the stigma that people with ADHD commonly face (and feel). Not only that, but these myths can stop people from accessing an assessment.

We have heard of doctors and psychologists saying, 'You can't have ADHD – you've got a degree!' or 'You can't have ADHD because you sat still during the consultation.' We even heard of a psychiatrist who said, 'Well, ADHD is very trendy nowadays, isn't it?'

Throughout wider society, as well as in healthcare and education, myths around ADHD have a real impact on our community. So, let's smash them into tiny little bits!

One of the most important but also infuriating things about science and research in general is that we don't really have a definite answer for anything for certain (scientists are usually the last people to 'know' anything!). Science isn't there to say something is definitely correct. Rather, it is a way of figuring out if an explanation is more likely to be correct than anything else we can think of at that moment.

Ironically, the idea of a 'scientific fact' is very rare. Uncertainty is a fundamental part of science and is key to changing our ideas and taking on new information as we get it. Unfortunately, that uncertainty is a magnet for bullshit.

With neurological disorders such as ADHD, this lack of clarity is particularly difficult. This is a relatively new field, so we often find studies with weak and conflicting evidence and gaps that need filling. This is where we see those myths and misunderstandings often gaining traction as people understandably try to fill the 'knowledge vacuum'. Hopefully, this chapter will give you a few more weapons to use if you hear some of this nonsense and decide you can't just let it go!

The media and ADHD

Both mainstream and wider media can be a fantastic resource for people who have (or think they might have) ADHD.

BUT...

Some of the 'less robust' journalism around ADHD often involves opinion pieces, informed by the authors' own biases and what they have read on the internet, and these can often be the prime source of these persistent and damaging myths. Articles such as 'I'm sorry, but all this

ADHD doesn't add up' (published in *The Sunday Times*[17]), 'I may not be a doctor ... but I'm almost certain you have ADHD' (*Guardian*[18]) and 'I'm calm and focused for this ADHD test', an apparently satirical piece (*The Times*[19]) according to the author, but one that clearly criticised a celebrity getting a diagnosis, offer easy clickbait and are designed to drive revenue for newspapers. But in the real world, these articles hurt people with ADHD.

Here are some of the common ADHD myths and what you need to know to bust them.

ADHD isn't real

This is one of the most repeated claims about ADHD, and it is pretty easy to see why this is. For most health conditions or diseases, you can usually take a simple test that gives you an unambiguous result. You can wee on a stick and find out if you are likely to have diabetes (at the doctors', not just any stick). But mental health conditions such as ADHD are different.

Diagnosis of pretty much all psychiatric disorders (including ADHD) rely on your subjective experience and your ability to describe your symptoms. For ADHD specifically, it also relies on evidence that you have had the symptoms since you were a child and for more than six months as an adult. Unfortunately, at the moment, there is no blood test, brain scan or reliable and objective test that enables you to point at somebody and say, 'Them, them! They have ADHD!' (Obviously, it shouldn't happen exactly like this. Even though we can smell our own.)

ADHD UNPACKED

This lack of a definitive assessment for diagnosis is enough for people to default to the position of ADHD not being a 'real' thing. But these people could equally apply the same rules to depression, anxiety or other psychiatric or neurodevelopmental conditions. These conditions also have subjective tests, based on questions that the patient is asked, but are (mostly) accepted as being real in society. It is also worth noting that these other psychiatric disorders weren't always accepted. The history of psychiatric medicine is littered with (often misogynist) abuse and neglect. We would even argue that if you hurt your leg, there is no definitive blood test to assess how much pain you are in.

Now, in medical terms, this lack of a blood test can be overcome. ADHD meets the standard criteria for a 'mental disorder' and is considered valid because:

a) well-trained professionals in a variety of settings and cultures agree on its presence or absence using well-defined criteria

and

b) the diagnosis of ADHD is useful for predicting additional problems that a patient may have, as well as future patient outcomes, response to treatment and other features that indicate a consistent set of causes for the disorder.[20]

On the other hand, it probably doesn't help that in 2010 psychiatrists were STILL arguing (even in the respected

MYTH-UNDERSTANDINGS!

British Medical Journal) whether adult ADHD was real, two years after it was officially recognised.

What we know from masses of research (many thousands of papers) is that there *are* clear genetic, anatomical and functional differences in the brains of people with ADHD compared to the brains of people without ADHD (on average). One of the problems with this is that it is really expensive to scan a brain and ADHD science hasn't been very well funded. Therefore many of these studies use very small populations of people.

You probably remember from school (or beyond if you are a science person) that the smaller the sample size, the less reliable that is for making generalisations to a whole community. Possibly more importantly, all of the people with ADHD are neurodiverse *within* that ADHD neurodivergent population. That means that our brains aren't all the same. And while we are more likely to have shared biological differences and shared behaviours, it isn't true that we all have every ADHD trait and it also doesn't mean that (for example) James's brain looks the same as Alex's brain. Or works as well!

As a scientific community, we are getting closer (though frustratingly slowly) to being able to point to an individual brain scan and say, 'That person is likely to have ADHD' (with their permission obviously, not just shouting it at strangers in the street). In the past couple of years, we have started to see more studies being published using larger population samples that show definable differences in the brains of people with ADHD compared to people without

ADHD. It is clearly very real, and we really hope that when we have an objective test, this will help to diffuse some of the ridiculous 'ADHD isn't real' talk.

ADHD in adults isn't 'a thing'

It probably doesn't help, but ADHD wasn't officially 'a thing' in adults in 2008, even though it clearly was 'a thing' in adults for the history of, well, adults (human adults, at least). The medical world is sometimes slower to catch up with the real world, and it seems that even though there were years of research about ADHD in adults prior to 2008, it took a while for this to filter into healthcare systems. It also took a long time for health organisations (who set the diagnostic rules for medical conditions) to agree that adults can have ADHD.

Now the medical community accept that adult ADHD is a recognised and well-documented disorder. ADHD *is not* limited to children; its symptoms can and often do persist into adolescence and adulthood (we would argue 'always' but that is a discussion for another time). While these symptoms may change or manifest themselves differently in adults compared to children, adult ADHD is a real and diagnosable neurological and behavioural disorder. If you prefer to think of it as a condition or simply a difference, that is, of course, absolutely fine. The medical side of referring to ADHD as a disorder is there to provide a platform for supporting people with the difficulties that come with it, not of 'medicalising' anyone who chooses a different term.

MYTH-UNDERSTANDINGS!

The myth that ADHD people are lazy

It is bad enough living with ADHD and spending years, sometimes decades, thinking that we are just lazy, useless or unreliable. When you see those newspaper articles, or get hurtful comments from friends and even family, suggesting that people with ADHD lack willpower, it just confirms what we often already think about ourselves. But people with ADHD aren't lazy, even when we haven't done something that appears to be a relatively simple job. Alex doesn't believe anyone is lazy, but we (as a society) need to spend more time working out what people are good at.

This issue with acting on things is because people with ADHD have what is called in psychology circles an 'intention–action gap'. What this means (possibly obviously) is that we intend to do things and then we don't do them. Or rather, we *can't* do them even if we want to (this isn't about willpower). There are a number of reasons for this. For many people with ADHD, the executive dysfunction of struggling to organise, motivate, prioritise and engage in tasks creates a big gap between what we intend to do and what we actually do. The brain has to combine 'planning a task' and 'wanting to do that task' to get it done. We have a gap when it comes to combining those. This is also called an 'intention deficit' and it is crippling. Not only because it creates problems doing the things we have to do (and even want to do), but it also creates feelings of worthlessness, embarrassment and shame and guilt.

While everybody, if they are honest, will admit that there are times when they want to 'do nothing', the burning shame of not being able to do something that you intend to do (and possibly have done before) is very real for people with ADHD. To suggest we don't engage in some tasks because we are lazy is ironically a lazy response to a real ADHD trait. Instead of just saying 'willpower', understanding why a task is difficult for us, what might help us see the reward in it and helping us to understand which bits are blocking us from doing (or even starting) a task, is much more useful than an unhelpful criticism that we lack willpower and are lazy.

When we are coaching people to do any task (for example, tidying a room), the blockage isn't laziness and usually isn't even the lack of motivation to tidy, but instead it is confusion about where to put the now-tidied stuff, for example. This is a lack of clarity on the process or a lack of that reward feeling for starting or finishing it.

We would advise ADHD people to write a 'DONE LIST'. That is a list of things they have done today or this week. It is often a bigger list than they think, but not always what they should have been doing. That isn't laziness; it is working with ADHD to get things done.

ADHD is caused by bad parenting

This is a big one. Research into the stigma of ADHD suggests that parents of children with ADHD often feel like (and often are) victims of societal stigma. This is particularly apparent for mothers of children with ADHD (for obvious reasons of 'cultural expectations').

Years of false information about the impact of parenting style on ADHD has led to the widely accepted view that

ADHD is caused by bad parenting. This is made worse by occasional (poorly designed) research studies, which might find there is a tenuous link between parenting style and ADHD (you can find anything if you go looking for it). Unfortunately, these types of studies often get press coverage that people inexplicably trust. Those papers almost always forget that ADHD is highly heritable from parents to children through their genes (see Chapter 2 on causes of ADHD).

It is important to note that extremely bad parenting, to the point of physical abuse or severe deprivation, may contribute as one of the environmental factors that trigger the genetic risk of developing ADHD. This is likely to be quite rare and isn't what people usually mean when they blame parents for their child's ADHD. The good news is that although parenting doesn't cause ADHD, healthy parenting strategies can play a crucial role in managing ADHD symptoms and supporting children with their ADHD. This might be as simple as asking children with ADHD when they are most able to focus on schoolwork or what would help them when they feel particularly physically uncomfortable and hyperactive.

All this modern technology causes ADHD

The 'mobile phone causing ADHD' myth is so ridiculous that we can deal with this in two paragraphs. ADHD was first described in medical texts in 1775, and in British medical texts in 1798.[21] We are pretty sure that mobile phones, tablets and games consoles weren't around during that time, or in the 1980s when ADHD came into public discourse. Apart from those massive brick-like phones that stockbrokers had in 80s films. You couldn't play *Farmville* on those though.

What we do know is that adults with ADHD are more likely to have smartphone addiction (or 'use-disorder' or 'maladaptive behaviour' if you don't like the word addiction for behavioural things). We are also more likely to spend increased time on smartphones. Additionally, children now have access to smartphones and apps that weren't available even ten years ago. None of this, however, provides even the slightest bit of evidence that mobile phone use causes ADHD. The idea that ALL of society is now less able to focus because of technological advances, smartphones and the internet is often quoted, but also not necessarily true (it might be) and it certainly isn't the same as an increase in ADHD. There is a lack of understanding of what ADHD is by some very basic units. Even this pervasive idea that our attention span is affected by technology is far more nuanced and, in some cases, isn't true at all.

ADHD is trendy so everyone's jumping on the bandwagon

It is easy to understand where this idea might have come from. Since the COVID-19 pandemic and associated lockdowns, many people have started to see information and thoughts on ADHD on social media platforms such as TikTok. More and more celebrities are announcing their diagnoses in the press. It is easy to see why people, who several years ago had no idea ADHD existed and now feel they are suddenly seeing it EVERYWHERE, might think, 'Where the hell did this come from? We didn't have this in my day!'

MYTH-UNDERSTANDINGS!

But they did have it in their day. The truth is that ADHD has been around for as long as humans have. The traits hang around in the population because having just a few of them is really quite useful (for everyone). If you have them too strongly or too many of them though, they become impairing (this is why ADHD traits in general can be broadly positive but ADHD itself isn't – too much of a good thing).

Following a podcast episode, we made ironic t-shirts with 'I have a defect of moral control' emblazoned on them. This statement came from one of the earliest terms for ADHD from paediatrician Sir George Frederic Still in 1902. Alongside those eighteenth-century papers, the idea of this being a new and 'trendy' bandwagon is clearly nonsense.

Finally, if ADHD is a trendy bandwagon, then it is the shittiest bandwagon ever. In some areas, it can take more than five years to get an assessment, you end up with loads of societal stigma, and all you get when you climb onto the bandwagon, if you are lucky, is some really weak speed. This isn't a bandwagon we can imagine many would want to jump on if they knew anything about it at all.

You can't be clever or have good grades if you have ADHD

While there is research showing that, *on average*, people with ADHD have poorer academic outcomes,[22] this doesn't mean that people with ADHD are by default less clever (they are not) or worse at learning. ADHD doesn't have to be a barrier to academic success! Instead, the way in which schools and universities are set up often puts barriers in place for people with ADHD to succeed.[23] Many schools and universities lack specialist knowledge in how to manage and support ADHD (not all schools and universities, it should be said – some are brilliant!). This lack of specialism often means they might mistakenly apply support strategies that work for other issues, such as dyslexia, without any evidence that those same strategies would help with ADHD in general.

Without blowing our own trumpets too much, we both managed to navigate school and university to obtain PhDs (although Alex claims James's PhD thesis was written in crayon). This doesn't make us especially clever or different to other people with (or without) ADHD, but James was fortunate to have a subject that he found rewarding and then focused on it. Alex didn't have the same experience and didn't have a healthy PhD experience.

For both of us though, the process of getting to this level of academic achievement came at a high cost, especially as we were diagnosed with ADHD as adults much later on. We achieved our qualifications despite a lack of ADHD support, which had (and continues to have) mental and physical health consequences. There is evidence that treating and managing ADHD in children improves academic performance, and this should be the opportunity that everyone is afforded.

Women don't have ADHD

One of the many systematic barriers to getting assessed, receiving a diagnosis or accessing support for women is

MYTH-UNDERSTANDINGS!

the very system that diagnoses ADHD itself. The diagnostic tests for ADHD (which are still used today) were developed using male children. This is highly likely to discriminate against girls, especially in the inattentive symptom list.

This discrimination is compounded by the fact that boys and girls with ADHD often don't act in the same way (on average). Boys can often, but not always, be more externally hyperactive and behaviourally challenging and overtly behave differently to other children. Girls with ADHD, on the other hand, are more likely than boys to be more anxious and 'daydreamy' (this word in itself is discriminatory because it is used negatively and more often against girls, rather than as a symptom of struggling with attention), and internalise their symptoms to fit in with society's expectations of what a girl or woman should be.

This is an issue that affects everyone, not just women. Alex, for example, showed almost all of the symptoms of ADHD traditionally associated with the female side (and still does). James was somewhere in the middle.

It is generally accepted that the ADHD test was designed more around symptoms seen in boys and also doesn't pick up the symptoms as well in girls. It is perhaps blatantly obvious then that the result of this was a dramatic difference in the number of boys diagnosed with ADHD compared to the number of girls, with roughly five times as many boys diagnosed as girls.[24]

The discrimination doesn't stop there because men and women with ADHD can often present differently. Evidence suggests that socially visible hyperactivity and impulsivity traits are more likely to be found in males (probably for cultural reasons) and more inattentiveness is seen in females. This also means it can be harder for women to get a diagnosis, even though the diagnostic levels between men and women are roughly equal.[25]

ADHD and the intersections of society

There are similar challenges for other groups with ADHD, including those from ethnic minorities, cisgendered or non-heteronormative people, and those with limited access to healthcare. There is very little research published in some of these groups, and this amplifies the discrimination that healthcare systems often have in place.

A huge American study of nearly a quarter of a million people found that Asian, Black and Hispanic children were significantly less likely to be diagnosed with ADHD compared with White children.[26] Other studies have shown that people from the LGBTQ+ community are more likely to experience a mental health disorder including ADHD,[27] and adults with ADHD are more likely to express variation from gender conformity.[28]

There are many reasons for this. But from a support perspective, that is yet another structural barrier to overcome, when ADHD by itself creates a very difficult set of social and personal challenges.

We are, without question, not the main people anybody should be asking about pretty much any intersection. We can and will talk about statistics and science from fantastic (and not so fantastic) research. But from an expert opinion perspective, we think the best thing our unearned privileged status in society gives us is to listen to people with actual lived experience.

ADHD is just an excuse for poor behaviour and choices

Believe us, if ADHD were a choice, no one would be choosing the superpower of losing their keys five times a day. But many people still feel that having ADHD is somehow an excuse to play a 'get out of jail free' card. In an interview with Times Radio in 2023, James was asked, 'Are we not just pathologising a lack of resilience in people?' In a nutshell, this is what many people think: 'I can do that stuff, why can't they? They're not trying hard enough.'

ADHD is an absolutely valid reason – not an excuse. No one wants to be able to do the things we often struggle with more than we want to, but our brains are just wired differently, making the executive functions that help us engage with day-to-day life more challenging. By accepting that we have a reason for being this way, instead of excusing ourselves, it enables us to explore new ways of getting things done in a more ADHD-friendly way. Would anyone who ever said this also say that people with physical disabilities were just making excuses? We don't think so.

ADHDers are more creative

In a moment of creativity, somebody came up with the word 'ADHDer'. We are not sure if we like it. It might seem odd

ADHD UNPACKED

that we are trying to dispel a myth that apparently claims something positive about ADHD.

The first thing to say is that we think creativity isn't some innate ADHD trait, but it is a fundamental human trait. We are always looking for a positive lens, but without evidence that positivity can end up being toxic (or inspiration porn) and actually create an unfair sense of shame and guilt. So it is important to provide a balanced evidence-based approach to all these ideas of what ADHD is (and isn't).

A little bit of evidence suggests that some adults with ADHD are better at some types of creative thinking than their ordinary counterparts. However, this isn't particularly strong or high-quality evidence, and we think these studies are usually describing the reward-seeking nature of people with ADHD more than higher levels of creativity itself. For example, people with ADHD thinking up lots of ideas for treats or cash in a short-term experiment. This is sometimes called divergent thinking, and a few studies have found small differences between people with ADHD and people without ADHD.

Some of the other studies on ADHD creativity are based on simply asking people with ADHD if they think they are creative thinkers. This tends to lead to a lot of people saying, 'Yes.' The main issue with the 'asking people how they feel' approach to research is that it really doesn't work and can be incredibly weak evidence, especially when you have people with poor metacognition skills.

Other studies have at least tried to apply a more objective test for creative thinking. This is very tricky to do,

76

partly because you have to design the experiments, but also because no one seems to be able to agree on what creativity is in the first place. The objective tests are more scientific, but an example might be paying children money to draw as many monsters as they can think of on a piece of paper. While in these experiments those ADHD children might draw more monsters than average children, that is very hard to recreate or sustain outside of an experiment, and it is also hard to prove that this is true creativity rather than a higher level of motivation. For example, in a one-off experiment, the ADHD children might be more likely to feel considerable reward from the money and the excitement of doing a research study for the first time. That doesn't necessarily make them more creative and certainly doesn't make it a consistent element off their personality.

Similarly, tasks that for most people are simple (such as basic admin and housework), people with ADHD can find overwhelming and stressful. This can lead to them to create new and interesting ways to get round existing challenges. Learning how to be creative to deal with problems that other people don't normally face isn't the same as a person with ADHD having some natural-born gift for creativity. Rather, we had to try different creative things because the 'typical' way of working wasn't effective at all.

People with ADHD probably aren't born more innately creative. The 'strengths' of ADHD are spread as equally across the ADHD community as across any community. Some of us are creative thinkers. Some of us are entrepreneurial. Some of us are tall. But we don't say people with ADHD are taller. Like height, creativity is a human trait, not an ADHD trait.

ADHD is overdiagnosed

The final myth in our list is the unhelpful belief that too many people are diagnosed with ADHD and it is too easy to get a diagnosis. This is particularly galling for anyone who was blocked from a referral, misdiagnosed, stuck on an endless waiting list or simply baffled by the forms, admin and confusion of getting an ADHD diagnosis in the first place.

We have seen many media attempts to frame this as a reactionary clickbait over the years, partly because the massive levels of underdiagnosis are being slowly rectified.[29] What may look like some kind of diagnosis explosion is actually a backlog due to years of neglect. When you look at the data from a centralised health service (such as the NHS in the UK), you can see that less than 0.5% are routinely prescribed ADHD medication (and that figure is a lot lower for adults). This suggests that we are still very far from both diagnosing and certainly treating adults with ADHD.

Learning from these myths

There may be some truth to some of these myths. We are always on the lookout for positives of ADHD. So, even though there isn't a lot of evidence that we were born with special powers such as extra creativity or lightning speed, it might be that growing up with ADHD leads to a sort of 'superpower' in a different way. We had to spend all of those formative years living and dealing with the impairments of ADHD and figuring out creative ways to succeed. Learning from that experience could definitely be an advantage

MYTH-UNDERSTANDINGS!

(although it requires privilege and luck in life too – but we will take it). Not fitting in can also provide you with a different perspective, which is why companies benefit from having ADHD folk in their organisations. It isn't the mythical superpowers that matter, but the benefit and empathy of our lived experience.

Many of the myths and misunderstandings about ADHD (such as the creativity one) are done out of positive intent. There are also many forces for good advocating for evidence-based information and dispelling these myths. Charities and organisations such as CHADD,[30] Healthline[31] and our charity ADHDadultUK provide evidence-based information that can help to fight the spread of these myths and to improve societal understanding of ADHD. We should probably point out that much of this work is done by Mrs AuDHD – who inexplicably agreed to marry James – as well as incredible volunteers and trustees.

SUMMARY

There are many persistent and damaging myths surrounding ADHD that are very unhelpful for the ADHD community. The lack of understanding and social acceptance of adult ADHD, which is informed by these myths, leads to stigma. These myths are mostly very easy to rebut with evidence, and it is important to take this opportunity to address them. With improved understanding of ADHD comes reduced myth and stigma.

We will be looking at the idea that ADHD comes with innate advantages and strengths rather than being a disorder that has required a new set of skills to overcome. This discourse is very difficult to combat because it feels positive at first glance but can lead to a problem receiving support. Overcoming challenges is a fantastic thing and can definitely be seen as a superpower, but that shouldn't be mistaken for some magical or supernatural set of skills we have. For reasons that will hopefully become clear in the next chapter, we call this 'difference': Batman vs. Superman.

CHAPTER 5

ADHD isn't a superpower for everybody

The question of whether ADHD is purely a disorder or some kind of evolutionary advantage causes much controversy within the ADHD community. Whichever side of the fence you sit on, we won't try to persuade you that ADHD is or isn't a superpower, and we certainly won't make you feel that other people can 'handle ADHD' better than you. Instead, what we *will* do is explain why ADHD isn't a superpower for everybody.

We need to reiterate that we know a positive outlook is fundamental for a healthy life with ADHD. It is equally important to emphasise that *acknowledging* any condition, disorder or disability isn't the same as *wallowing*. Accepting a difficult situation and adopting a positive lens is often the best way to move forward. It isn't a fight between two positions. Everyone with ADHD, regardless of their perception of ADHD, can improve things by saying, 'This is real. what steps can I take now?'

ADHD isn't a superpower for everyone

This is important to understand because it doesn't mean being negative. In fact, having a positive lens is one of the most powerful ways of learning to live with ADHD. Seeing yourself and the disorder as wholly negative is damaging. People with ADHD can do (almost) anything with the right support. However, it is common to take this positive message and assume that everyone born with ADHD has 'mystical superpowers' that enable us to achieve more than ordinary non-ADHD people. This is toxic positivity. It isn't helpful nor is it a positive lens.

What is toxic positivity?

When the good, powerful and famous have ADHD, there is often a tendency to assume that they have achieved *because* of ADHD, rather than sheer hard work and talent (and a little bit of luck). We have even read research papers where rich people with ADHD were asked if their success was due to ADHD, and they said it was. But how would they know if it wasn't due to ADHD? It is impossible to tell, as there isn't a 'non-ADHD' version of themselves to compare anything to.

We have also lost count of the number of times we have heard apparently positive aspects of ADHD being described by successful people, such as:

'Having lots of energy is a good thing.'

'Being distracted and impulsive means you get to an idea quicker.'

'*You can think out of the box.*'

'*You can make more connections.*'

Ironically, people often say that these are ADHD traits because they are being humble about their personal talents. Humility often appears as a result of the effect of ADHD on self-esteem and self-awareness. It can be very difficult for adults with ADHD to show confidence in our talents and pride in achievements and hard work because we spend our lives feeling that we can't do some of the simplest tasks that most people find easy. So, it can feel less arrogant to 'blame' ADHD for these skills.

Why does it matter?

Even if you ignore the fact that there is little evidence for many of these perceived, innate qualities being higher in the average person with ADHD, this view suggests to the millions of people for whom their ADHD is a daily struggle, that if they had just applied themselves, they would also be successful. This can be really painful.

Describing ADHD as a series of creative and energetic advantages that you should somehow be tapping into doesn't speak to the general experience of living with ADHD for most people. Especially those without access to diagnosis, treatment, support and financial advantage. This is a more toxic form of positivity.

But, what about talent and hard work? Toxic positivity ignores these qualities (as well as privilege) in a noble attempt to be inspirational when, in fact, these can have the opposite effect. For example, if you are able to afford a personal assistant, or work in a role in which you are assigned a personal assistant, a lot of the organisational admin that can be challenging to deal with if you have ADHD will be taken care of. This then enables you to focus on things you find more rewarding, and to become really good at it.

Equally, if you have a career in which you find the core elements are rewarding for you personally, you will likely be more able to engage with the aspects of that career that lead to success, and then, by working hard on it, may become successful. For example, we often hear that people think careers in creative arts and sports are more likely to lead to ADHD success. That may be true for people who can access the training, have the talent and work hard and, crucially, who find that specific field highly interesting, but it doesn't mean everyone with ADHD will be better at that.

Using the example of these successful people, who have had the right support and environment in which to thrive, can lead many people with ADHD to feel that not only are they struggling in life, but they can't even exploit their own mental health condition properly. Internalising the idea that if you aren't a creative and successful genius then you are not doing ADHD properly, isn't true, and nor is it helpful.

If we don't take into account talent, hard work and luck, we can make poor conclusions based on a view called 'success bias' or 'survivor bias'. Survivor bias is a logical error of concentrating on people who achieved visible successes while overlooking those who didn't. This is a poor and

ADHD ISN'T A SUPERPOWER FOR EVERYBODY

inaccurate way to understand people with ADHD. Asking for the reasons for success only from highly successful people with ADHD will obviously skew the perception of ADHD. Survivor bias can be like trying to predict next week's lottery numbers by asking previous winners of the lottery. Trying to learn from survivor bias doesn't take into account the many other factors (such as luck) or barriers to success.

If we also look at this from a scientist's perspective, ideas around innate (naturally present from birth) ADHD superpowers don't appear to be true. For example, the belief that we have 'more energy' often comes from observing adults with ADHD in a highly charged environment, in which people see us being energetic and motivated and assume that this is a permanent state. It doesn't take into account the rest we need, the burnout and the heavy emotional cost of these energetic periods.

If you look at the data, one study demonstrated more fatigue in people with ADHD than those without ADHD.[32] It is more likely that the perception we have more energy is based on people watching us in a new or exciting environment with lots of people, or it is only looking at people who are able to do the tasks they find (currently) particularly motivating. That isn't representative of how most days work for most people with ADHD.

Another common ADHD 'superpower' is this idea that we make lots of connections that others don't make. We are never entirely sure what people mean when they say 'connections' or that we 'think outside of the box', but it seems to allude to some form of creativity that we discussed in the myths section of Chapter 4. This is often known as 'divergent thinking', another trait often linked in higher levels to ADHD, but when we looked at a range of studies on creativity, the results show that this just isn't correct. We are in broadly the same range as everyone else.

It shouldn't be (but sometimes is) controversial to say that creativity is a human trait, rather than an ADHD trait. It kind of defines what humanity is. We could only find a handful of studies suggesting one or two elements of higher creativity, but most studies don't find any significant difference in creativity between ADHD groups and the rest of the population. Even our previous example of paying children with ADHD to draw more monsters is hard to interpret as a direct measure of creativity. Was it a repeatable experiment? Possibly not. Is it creativity that drives the child or the reward? What if they had to do it every day? We don't think this proves a long-term measure of innately high creativity compared to say, a measure of short-term motivation in an experimental setting.

Bafflingly, the American ADHD magazine *ADDitude*[33] published an article from their own editorial team with the sentence, 'The positives of ADHD are numerous and mighty – creativity, empathy, and tenacity, just to name a few.' The challenge there is finding any evidence whatsoever to back up those statements, especially as 'asking people with ADHD' doesn't take into consideration that people with ADHD (including us) often lack self-awareness compared to the general population AND are more likely to overestimate their abilities.

We laugh when told that we are particularly resilient and tenacious, for example. We think that 'resilient and tenacious'

ADHD ISN'T A SUPERPOWER FOR EVERYBODY

refers to the concept of not giving up, so this implies that people with ADHD aren't doing this. In our experience, anyone with ADHD and an attic has filled it with the skeletons of long-dead hobbies that we assumed we would be committing to for the rest of our lives. In our case, Alex has a surfboard and rock-climbing equipment, while James has three thousand guitars and a typewriter.

This is funny because in addition to tenacity requiring us to sustain attention, famously a key challenge for an attentional disorder, one of the DSMV criteria is, 'Often does not follow through on instructions and fails to finish schoolwork, chores, or duties in the workplace (e.g., starts tasks but quickly loses focus and is easily side-tracked).' Emotional resilience and emotional dysregulation are also quite difficult to align in many of us.

Back to ADHD as a superpower. If we are going to call it that, we want to make a request that it is described as Batman rather than Superman. Superman was born with superpowers. He could fly, he had laser eyes and (we haven't checked this) he could somehow make time go backwards by spinning the planet the wrong way round (that doesn't feel like how time works).

Batman, on the other hand, wasn't born with special powers. He was born with privilege: specifically, billions of pounds and a loving family (and a butler). However, he also had to face challenges that most people don't in life (in his case, being orphaned rather than ADHD). This meant he had to develop skills that other people didn't or couldn't develop, and he had the talent and tenacity to develop them.

What we are suggesting here is that most perceived ADHD advantages develop as a response to *living with* ADHD. We have to find new ways of thinking, not because we are innately more creative but because the usual methods that seem simple for most people are often difficult for people with ADHD. We also like to invite people to think about whether luck and privilege played a small part, *as well as* hard work and talent. When we share that privilege, we can reduce the barriers to success for everyone.

When we talk about privilege in an ADHD context, we are not just talking about having a butler (although that would solve a lot of our ADHD problems). We are talking about a stable upbringing, an emotionally safe family and school, and being born in a culture where treatment and diagnosis are available. We know that the less fortunate someone is in life, the more likely they are to face difficulties due to their ADHD. This is unfairness and inequality, not a lack of effort.

We also think that it is a bit unfair to expose celebrities with ADHD as ambassadors when they are early in their journey. This is a complex and changing time, and asking them to be spokespeople for an entire community with a complex neurological condition has led to unfortunate statements that get a lot of airtime and cause quite a bit of damage and misinformation (someone in the media recently announced that ADHD was caused by sugary drinks). We want to remind everyone that sharing your experiences is always positive, but you can be an expert for your *own* ADHD without generalising for the rest of us.

SUMMARY

It is vital to look at your ADHD and ask, 'How can I be a success with this, not against it?' A positive lens is proven to improve our mental health and drive success. You can acknowledge the challenges of ADHD without having to invent a set of advantages we are born with that don't appear to be based on anything but our own thoughts about our individual skills, talents and ADHD. Your ADHD isn't the same as anyone else's. In all cases, though, we need support to fly!

If the world assumes that ADHD (wrongly) solely offers innate advantages, this can have the counterproductive effect of making people think, 'Why do I need support if ADHD is such a superpower?' We need to acknowledge the many challenges of untreated, unsupported ADHD as a starting point for success.

This is just one of the reasons why it is so important to keep a positive lens with ADHD but also to avoid the idea that it is some kind of innate advantage. The superpower myth can lead to a reduction in support and increase the stigma of having ADHD for the people who don't feel highly creative and successful. The internalisation of this stigma can also create barriers to getting a diagnosis of ADHD in the first place.

If an ADHD diagnosis is seen as unnecessary (or negative), this will seriously risk people not getting the support they need. We all know the diagnosis itself is a minefield, with challenges of executive function, communication and access to health services. In the next chapter, we will look at that diagnosis process and how it differs across countries and systems.

CHAPTER 6

ADHD diagnosis

In this chapter, we will explain how ADHD is typically diagnosed (in most places in the world). There may be a few differences because of different health systems, laws and uses of words such as 'disorder', 'disability' and 'diagnosis'. We will point out where it gets a bit messy (spoiler alert: it is everywhere as ADHD diagnosis is an absolute minefield). There are also some subtle differences in how ADHD is diagnosed in adults compared to children, although the core elements of diagnosing adults and children with ADHD (such as the list of symptoms) are very similar (despite the fact that they probably shouldn't be).

What can people actually get diagnosed with?

We have already discussed in Chapter 1 that there are (currently) three medically accepted flavours of ADHD. We know 'flavours' is a strange choice of word, but we got bored with writing 'type' all the time. 'Presentation' is the official terminology. These flavours of ADHD are:

- inattentive presentation

- hyperactive-impulsive presentation

- combined presentation.

The estimates vary, but around 50–70 per cent of all adults appear to have the triple whammy, which (as the name suggests) combines both the inattentive-type ADHD (formally ADD) and the hyperactive-impulsive type ADHD (having this last one on its own only affects a very small number of people and may even be a different disorder altogether).

This decision or diagnosis of your ADHD type can't, in most cases, be made by your GP (or family doctor) BUT in many countries (unless you have private medical care), you may have to approach them first to get referred to someone who can diagnose you. We strongly advise having some notes on your history and information prepared in advance of that first conversation.

How do they decide if you are diagnosable?

There is no blood test (or any other objective measure) for any psychiatric condition including ADHD. This can give fuel to the people who (wrongly) think ADHD isn't real. It can get a bit frustrating when people say that, especially when they don't deny the existence of other mental health conditions because, ironically, ADHD is the one with the strongest evidence of a clear biology.

For now, we are left with a diagnosis that is (at least partly) subjective based on who assesses you, as well as the information you are able to provide. The word 'able' is key, as there are many barriers to accessing personal history. In both of our cases, for example, we just weren't paying attention as kids for some reason, and now can't remember. This need for memories and evidence from your childhood obviously isn't ideal and can lead to both false positives (where you don't have ADHD but you do get a diagnosis) and false negatives (where you do have ADHD but don't get a diagnosis). At the moment, though, it is the best we have. OK, not the best. It is what we have.

Although there isn't a definite medical consensus on the questions and symptoms that make up this subjective test for ADHD, most psychiatrists turn to what we refer to as the 'Big Boring American Book of Mental Health Conditions'. 'We' being the two of us, obviously, and not the broader 'we' of proper grown-ups.

This book's more accurate name is the unnecessarily long *Diagnostic and Statistical Manual of Mental Disorders; 5th edition* (or 'DSMV').[34] It is published by the American Psychiatric Association (APA). Incidentally, the APA made the (probably wise) decision in 1892 to change their name from the 'Association of Medical Superintendents of American Institutions for the Insane'. Their DSMV book has a dual purpose. Firstly, it lists and describes the different types and classes of psychiatric disorders (called taxonomy). Secondly, it is used by doctors as a diagnostic tool to see if we have ADHD at all.

The fifth edition of the DSM was published in 2013, and we are eagerly awaiting the next version. There was a small revision in March 2022 (DSM-5-TR) and this is the edition that most doctors use as their guide. You might also see people refer to a different guide, called the International Classification of Diseases (ICD), produced by the World Health Organization (WHO) and currently on the eleventh edition (ICD-11).[35] The specifics of the ICD-11 for mental health conditions are discussed in this paper.[36]

In the UK, the NHS officially use the ICD-11 (although most of the doctors we speak to use the DSMV). The main difference is that the DSMV says you need five out of the nine listed symptoms to qualify for an adult ADHD diagnosis (six out of nine in children), but the ICD-11 just says 'several', which is reassuringly ambiguous. Regardless of which big boring book you use, the symptoms are suspiciously similar. The DSM and ICD lists of ADHD symptoms are incredibly similar, and the difference really is just one for the ADHD nerds, so you might want to look that up if you are that kind of person.

What is a typical process of 'ADHD diagnosis'?

The pathway to getting an ADHD diagnosis almost always requires a number of steps, with at least two visits/conversations with a trained expert (the assessor). This is one reason (along with underfunding) why the waiting list for an ADHD diagnosis can be months or even years, especially where there is a national health service rather than private healthcare system. Many people feel pushed into getting

ADHD DIAGNOSIS

private healthcare, which has its own potential drawbacks and risks. We will discuss this later in this chapter.

These conversations are usually with a doctor (but not always) and will probably be based around those DSMV criteria. However, this should also include a thorough conversation about you as a person. 'Should' being the keyword because the quality of this experience varies a lot. Ideally, this conversation should include your current situation but also memories of you as a child, even drawing on feedback from employers, family and friends, if possible. It can also include old school reports, memories from anyone who knew you as a child and, in fact, anything else you can prepare in advance to explain things. The steps should include:

1. a medical, psychological and social assessment of you – this has to be a conversation that talks about the behaviours and symptoms in the different parts of everyday life

2. a full developmental and psychiatric history from early childhood

3. observer reports and assessment of your mental state.

This isn't always the case. For example, Alex was never asked to provide observer reports at any point in his diagnosis. It is also quite common to have an initial meeting with someone on the mental health team to discuss with you where to find this information. Many people aren't told that this isn't the actual meeting where they make a decision on your diagnosis. That is a common example of the barrier to

95

getting a diagnosis for neurodivergent people, struggling with understanding these sorts of processes.

Then, there is usually the 'actual' consultation in which the expert assessor decides you have ADHD (and if you have got this far, it usually does mean you have ADHD) along with which type.

What are the behaviours and symptoms of the different ADHD types?

Inattentive-type ADHD (formerly ADD)

In order to be diagnosed with inattentive-type ADHD, most diagnosing professionals would start with that 'assessment' conversation. They are highly likely to base the diagnosis on those common symptoms in the DSMV (and pretty similar for the ICD-11) book. They also are looking for evidence that those symptoms:

- cause a sufficient impairment in functioning specifically due to those symptoms of inattention

- lead to those impairments in more than at least two environments (home and work, for example)

- have been persistent since early childhood (usually under the age of twelve, but some people say under sixteen)

- aren't better explained by some other disorder – this is really controversial, bearing in mind that 80 per cent of adults with ADHD have at least one other disorder at the same time; James, for example,

ADHD DIAGNOSIS

has cyclothymia, a form of bipolar disorder, binge eating disorder, social phobia and many, many other coexisting conditions. It isn't a competition, but if it were he would probably be winning.

The first element is to confirm that there are AT LEAST five out of nine (six out of nine in children) from the following symptoms of inattention (that we also introduced in Chapter 1). These symptoms have to be considered 'severe', which means they are happening often or very often. This severity is the difference between that myth that we are 'all a bit ADHD' and someone who faces this all of the time and actually has ADHD.

DSMV INATTENTIVE TYPE ADHD SYMPTOMS

1. Often fails to give close attention to details or makes careless mistakes in schoolwork, at work, or with other activities.

2. Often has trouble holding attention on tasks or play activities.

3. Often does not seem to listen when spoken to directly.

4. Often does not follow through on instructions and fails to finish schoolwork, chores, or duties in the workplace (e.g. loses focus, gets sidetracked).

5. Often has trouble organising tasks and activities.

6. Often avoids, dislikes, or is reluctant to do tasks that require mental effort over a long period of time (such as schoolwork or homework).

7. Often loses things necessary for tasks and activities (e.g. school materials, pencils, books, tools, wallets, keys, paperwork, eyeglasses, mobile telephones).

8. Is often easily distracted.

9. Is often forgetful in daily activities.

We are not saying this is a good list. Given the chance, we would change many aspects of this (particularly the wording). For example, 'Often has trouble organising tasks and activities' excludes people crippled by anxiety to the point that they do anything to avoid disorganisation – they are still having 'trouble with organisation' but that might not appear so, unless they were asked about the cost of that level of organisation. We would prefer the criteria to look at the mental, emotional and physical cost of having to be organised. This is especially important for people with a cultural expectation of responsibility (often more typical for women).

To see why ADHD can be a serious challenge, we would suggest looking at any one of those criteria on the list and asking yourself, 'Is that going to cause a problem in school, university, at work and in a family?' In almost every case, the answer is going to be 'Yes'. ADHD can be a significant barrier to success in life. Many of the things on the list are taken for granted as 'good values' to have or 'normal, simple and easy' in society and yet we struggle with them daily.

ADHD DIAGNOSIS

Hyperactive-impulsive type ADHD (fewer than 10 per cent of people)

This second type of ADHD is less common and some-times reflects that the impulsivity symptoms aren't overt yet, but might be later on. To get diagnosed with hyperac-tive-impulsive-type ADHD, it is exactly the same process as above for inattentive-type ADHD, but the assessor will start with a different list of common symptoms (also taken from the DSMV or ICD-11). As with inattentive-type ADHD, the assessor will need to be confident that the symptoms:

- cause a sufficient impairment in functioning specifically due to those symptoms of hyperactivity/ impulsivity

- lead to those impairments in more than one environment (so home and work, for example)

- have been persistent since early childhood (under twelve years old)

- aren't better explained by some other disorder.

Again, the assessor will usually be looking for AT LEAST five out of nine (six out of nine in children) from the follow-ing symptoms of hyperactivity/impulsivity and that they are severe (happening 'often' or 'very often'):

DSMV HYPERACTIVE-IMPULSIVE TYPE
ADHD SYMPTOMS

1. Often fidgets with or taps hands or feet, or squirms in seat.

2. Often leaves seat in situations when remaining seated is expected.

3. Often runs about or climbs in situations where it is not appropriate (adolescents or adults may be limited to feeling restless).

4. Often unable to play or take part in leisure activities quietly.

5. Is often 'on-the-go' acting as if 'driven by a motor'.

6. Often talks excessively.

7. Often blurts out an answer before a question has been completed.

8. Often has trouble waiting their turn.

9. Often interrupts or intrudes on others (e.g. butts into conversations or games).

Again, we don't love these lists. We wish that the criteria in this group would include the phrase, 'Or really wants to', because we know the human cost of blocking those urges can be really high.

When Alex was masking at work (many years ago), he would bite his mouth until it bled to avoid oversharing, interrupting and blurting out thoughts in a meeting. This would mean that he didn't 'often' do those things on the list, but clearly that was still a huge problem. We would also really like a change to some of the infantilising language, such as the use of fidgeting for hyperkinetic disorder in the first symptom description.

Another issue are those mysterious value judgements such as 'talks excessively'. The decision of what 'too much' talking is has no universal agreement and is often based on the majority view. We would argue that 'talks too little' could be applied to many people who don't have ADHD, but it isn't in a manual of mental disorders. This is a phenomenon well known to the neurodivergent community – called 'neuronormativity'. Another example is how autistic people have been told for years that they don't 'make enough eye contact' despite no evidence of eye contact being effective for authenticity.

Combined type ADHD

It is probably no surprise that to get a combined-type ADHD diagnosis (like both of us), you need to qualify for BOTH of the above ADHD types.

The above lists are powerful indicators that someone has ADHD, but it isn't possible to just say 'yes' or 'no' from those lists alone (for good reason!). This is mainly because they could easily miss people with ADHD who didn't answer the questions properly, were comparing themselves to family (who are also highly likely to have ADHD traits) or, in James's case, because he got bored halfway through filling in the forms and answered 'not applicable', based on thinking he had enough symptoms. He still managed to get a strong seven out of nine on the bits he did fill in.

What that means is the bit of the diagnosis where you talk about your history and impairments is usually a way for a psychiatrist to 'fill in the gaps' to make a meaningful diagnosis. So, what does that conversation usually look like?

What is meant by a 'full developmental and psychiatric history from early childhood'?

Many people tell us that they worry about how to get evidence for developmental and psychiatric history from their early childhood. We have had many frantic conversations from people concerned that their parents aren't around or won't engage because they don't believe ADHD is real. We have heard from people who have no powerful memories of their own childhood, and many who have lost all of their school reports. This is unsurprisingly quite common. The 'ADHD tax' of having to pay a school or college several times for copies of lost exam result certificates is a real one. We have the perfect solution for this: we keep them in a box in the loft. Or in the office or under the bed or something. Can't remember.

If any of that resonates with you, DON'T PANIC. Our main advice is to do as much as you can. 'Perfect' is the enemy of good in this and almost all circumstances. Mental health professionals are trained to understand that ADHD includes organisational challenges. That is part of the disorder. We have heard of psychiatrists who claim they can't diagnose because they rigidly stick to needing a parental report or school report. Not common, but this can happen. Most ADHD assessors are used to speaking with people who might not have a colour-coded file of school reports from the last twenty years arranged in alphabetical order. (If you do have that type of file, don't worry, it doesn't make you a fraud. Many people with ADHD appear massively organised, and overcompensating for a life of inattention can be a coping strategy.)

Assessors are also aware that many people might not have access to this information due to the relationship they have with their parents (relationship breakdown is MORE common in ADHD families, so again this won't be a surprise). The aim here is for the assessor to get as much information as they can from you. It isn't to trap you into admitting you were a perfect and normal child and that you are fraudulently looking for an ADHD diagnosis, so you don't have to admit you're just bad at being an adult. If you can think back to any time when life seemed difficult for you, especially with things that (according to society) 'shouldn't be that difficult', write them down and note how that made you feel. That is what they are looking for.

ADHD is a disorder of brain development and doesn't appear out of nowhere in adults (this isn't a value judgement on our part, it is part of the diagnostic criteria). This is why the 'history' and childhood part is fundamental to think about when preparing for an assessment. However, most adults are seeking a diagnosis for a pressing reason (the pandemic blew many coping strategies out of the water, for example), and is why the final part of the conversation will be about your current situation in life.

Observer reports and assessment of the person's mental state

Again, this can be a source of stress. This conversation will involve questions about many of those symptoms and behaviours and how they affect you now, both at home and in the workplace (or education or whatever you do to fill your days). You will be asked about your relationships (personal and professional) and your 'less healthy' life choices (nothing you say will surprise them, believe us).

How those symptoms manifest is very different for different people, and how that affects your life also depends on your culture, gender, upbringing, personality, what you had for lunch, general life stress and a million other things. You are not in competition with anyone – just be honest about how it feels.

Our golden rule is: Don't assume you will be able to think and remember clearly in the middle of an emotional conversation with a psychiatrist. Try to prepare your thoughts in advance. Saying this, we know someone who was criticised in their assessment for 'turning to their crib sheet' to their psychiatrist – there are as many horror stories as there are positive ones!

Any level of preparation requiring advanced writing is both boring and unlikely if you have ADHD (unless you happen to be hyperfocusing, then you might have 200 pages about your life). One place to start might be the simple 'check-box' style questionnaires you can find online, and many of these are free. One example of this (called the ASRS) can be found by following this link: https://psychology-tools. com/adult-adhd-self-report-scale/.

When you look at these questions, and if you tick some of the examples, try writing them down in case you forget. We also advise talking it through with someone you trust so it feels like more of a fun game rather than an admin task.

Checklist for preparing for your ADHD diagnosis

1. Have I done the thing they have asked me to on the letter?

2. Have I asked someone to read through my forms?

3. Have I given examples from my childhood at school and at home?

4. Have I given examples from my current life at home and out in the world?

5. Have I filled in a free online ADHD symptom question sheet?

Common questions you may want to ask about getting diagnosed

It is difficult to explain the diagnosis process that fits every-one and every system. Everyone has different experiences and questions about their own circumstances. While we can't anticipate every question, we often get asked the following common questions about the diagnostic process.

I think I have ADD. Why doesn't ADD exist anymore?

This is just a naming issue to make things clearer for medical treatment. The official name changed from ADD in the eighties, but is still used, particularly in America. The research currently states that ADHD without apparent hyperactivity isn't a separate condition with different treatment; you just present slightly differently with your ADHD. Many people still refer to their own inattentive-type ADHD as 'ADD' and should be respected. We would caution against telling other people they 'have ADD' unless they do first.

How do you know if these symptoms have a significant negative effect on your life?

This is part of the subjective element of ADHD. It isn't the same for everyone and is one of the ways people unfairly criticise ADHD as a 'lack of resilience'. Examples could include losing a job, alcohol (or substance) use disorder (AUD and SUD), relationship breakdowns, criminality, driving problems, a lack of promotion due to inappropriate behaviour, and lots of other things.

Of course, this is never black and white – you don't always know 'what might have been' – and it is hard to know if your impairment is worse than an average person's. If you have anyone in your life you could ask safely without getting upset, this would be a great place to start. This isn't always simple, though, and you need a good friend to answer honestly. This is important; so many people report to us that they feel fraudulent as they have no history of addiction, mental health problems or relationship issues. In many cases, this is because they are unaware of them.

Why do they ask if these symptoms have ALWAYS been there?

Once those criteria have been discussed, the clinician then has to make a series of decisions. The first one being: Is this a consistent thing throughout the life of the person in front of them?

It is (from a medical perspective) not considered possible for ADHD to suddenly appear in an adult. ADHD is a neurodevelopmental disorder caused by a difference in how your brain develops from early childhood. If you absolutely didn't have ADHD-like symptoms as a child, then it is HIGHLY unlikely that you would get a diagnosis of ADHD. This doesn't mean you aren't struggling, or it isn't as serious. It could be (for example) that you had some kind of head injury. This would also need treatment and therapy but tailored differently.

We are aware that the experiences of adults can be markedly different to their childhoods (hormonal changes during menopause, the absence of previously supportive parental structures, etc.). Despite this, evidence suggests that for the majority of people, the ability to compensate for these traits as a child would rule out a diagnosis of ADHD because ADHD is partly the lack of ability to compensate in the first place. An example of a child who might have compensated for ADHD would be an almost unheard-of level of school and social support in pretty much every environment of their life. While not impossible, this isn't a common experience. It is one of the elements of ADHD itself. We face quite a lot of 'feedback' for explaining this online, despite not necessarily agreeing with this diagnostic rule.

Why must these symptoms be seen in more than one area of your life?

This is similar to the reason why clinicians need ADHD symptoms to have been present from childhood. Many of the symptoms could be caused by something else. For example, a particularly difficult working environment could trigger concentration problems, boredom, distraction and emotional dysregulation. However, this might not always be your experience – for example, you might find concentrating at school fine, but not at home. Or, say working brings this out in you, but you didn't have these same issues navigating school, this may be something else and an ADHD diagnosis and treatment would be unhelpful.

A couple of issues with this include the difference between 'impairment' and 'ADHD trait'. The 'at least two environments' doesn't have to involve equal levels of impairment. If your family was happily chaotic, for example, the 'problems' doing normal tasks may not have been 'problems' for your family. The question is more about whether you had a problem doing them at all (not whether people minded). ADHD traits themselves can be exacerbated from time to time in ADHD adults, but they don't come and go completely.

Another issue is that ADHD isn't a lack of focus, but instead is a problem choosing what to focus on (and for how long). Many people, especially those who have coped by using their so-called 'hyperfocus' in their professional lives, can appear to find concentrating less problematic. Both Alex and James have done this. For James, that includes editing podcasts; for Alex, it is mainly thinking of ways to infuriate James on a daily basis. The key here is to explore how you are outside of your special interests (whatever they are). Some ADHD accountants might find their work absolutely absorbing and seem fine, but how are they with tasks that *aren't* interesting to them?

What do they mean, 'Is there anything else that could explain these symptoms?'

This is a tricky one. There are many psychiatric, social or medical conditions that could cause many of the symptoms of ADHD. These could include brain injury, PTSD, menopause, stress and anxiety, and bipolar disorder. It is important that a psychiatrist considers what else could be causing these symptoms and decides if the ADHD diagnosis is appropriate.

We think this should be far more flexible, since more than 80 per cent of people with ADHD have at least one other mental health condition. This means that (for example) a diagnosis of anxiety COULD explain some of the ADHD symptoms but equally could be a second condition.

Who can diagnose someone with ADHD?

Even within a single country, this isn't a simple question. There is a general agreement that, for the most part, this should be a psychiatrist (a doctor qualified in mental health diagnosis and treatment). Having said that, there are non-medical practitioners who are more than qualified and legally entitled to diagnose and treat people with ADHD. They might include clinical psychologists (usually not a medical doctor) and other mental health practitioners (e.g. advanced mental health nurse practitioners). For children in the UK, a specialist team is embedded in the school system, for whom the diagnosis is accepted by the NHS and enables a further route to treatment. Educational support for ADHD varies widely from country to country and even within local boundaries.

In the UK, the NHS tends to interpret the National Institute for Health and Care Excellence (NICE) guidelines as someone who has at least graduate qualifications in a health-related discipline and a current registration (or accreditation) with the main UK medical professional bodies (typically this means the General Medical Council, the Health and Care Professions Council or the Nursing and Midwifery Council). This is the bare minimum and isn't an automatic measure of competence for an ADHD assessment without 'appropriate skills and training in ADHD assessment and diagnosis'. Every country has different rules on this.

After that, it starts to get a bit grey and, in some cases, downright immoral with unscrupulous companies and individuals taking thousands of pounds to tell you that you have ADHD but with no real qualifications to make that

ADHD DIAGNOSIS

decision in a meaningful way. If you are looking for a diagnosis that means any medical doctor would be confident to give you a prescription for treatment, make sure you ask in advance if your planned route of diagnosis fits within their expectations. The different levels and credibility of a 'diagnosis' are incredibly frustrating and a minefield for anyone, least of all those of us who struggle with the admin and research needed to organise this kind of task.

What about private diagnoses?

Getting a diagnosis of ADHD through a private clinic is much faster than with a national health service (certainly in the UK). Privately, you can expect to be diagnosed in as little as two weeks) but there are significant costs attached. If you access a private diagnosis (or can only do that), be aware that you are usually going to pay for all of the steps, including:

- the initial consultation (not typically with your diagnosing professional but to give you the forms to fill in)

- the professional consultation (to discuss those forms and other areas with you)

- the cost of a medical professional who can prescribe your medication – this also includes checking how you react to it, changing the dose, etc.

- the cost of the medication itself at the pharmacy (it will be prescribed privately so you can't pick it up like an NHS prescription)

- the cost of a discharge consultation.

A private diagnosis is, in our experience (at the time of writing), going to be around £1,000, and it could end up being significantly higher than that. We are also aware that some private diagnoses don't include any treatment and probably wouldn't speed up your access to treatment through your national health service. They can be useful to access employer/university support and reasonable adjustments but be clear on what it is you need from a private diagnosis.

If you are in a country with private health insurance, the cover for ADHD depends on the country and in many cases the individual insurance company, so check and double-check the fine print.

In the UK, if you want to go to the NHS for continued care after your private diagnosis, you first have to check that your GP is willing to accept the 'Shared Care Agreement' that your private psychiatrist will pass to them. Some GPs don't engage with this as it is a professional courtesy, not an obligation. Other countries with centralised healthcare systems (such as Australia, Canada, New Zealand and Norway) all have their own rules for moving to national health support after a private diagnosis. For countries with a more embedded private health insurance system, this is dependent on the insurance companies' specific small print and both national and local rules on ADHD support.

I was diagnosed by my university, school or college. Will a psychiatrist prescribe ADHD treatment based on that?

Although there is no clear answer to this question within the UK, and certainly not globally, it is safest to assume that this might not be the case. It is typically a fantastic educational institute or company that will support reasonable adjustments by trusting your word, though we want that to be standard. We also know that some of these organisations even fund their own educational specialists to help you understand your possible learning needs and challenges (likely including ADHD).

The danger is that we have heard from many people who thought their educational establishment supporting their self-diagnosis of ADHD was enough to qualify them for medical treatment from a clinician. This then caused huge disappointment (and a long wait for treatment) when that clinician insisted on sending them back to the referral queue. Confusion around institutional support and who can provide a formal and widely accepted medical diagnosis is exactly why we need clearer rules on diagnosis and treatment.

I have my ADHD diagnosis, so what next?

A significant majority (probably over 90 per cent) of people who realise that ADHD might be a fit for them (they often do A LOT of research about it), and then get a referral for ADHD, do meet the diagnostic criteria and receive a diagnosis of ADHD. This shouldn't be that surprising as it is a big list of things that most people don't find too tricky in life. Trying to explain to most people about some of our very basic challenges can feel like explaining *Love Island* to Abraham Lincoln. They might understand most of what you are saying but they are likely to think you are making it up.

Once you have your diagnosis, what happens next? Some people don't need anything, the diagnosis can itself suffice. Saying this, many clinicians tell us that a few months after a diagnosis, many people decide they might need additional support. There are no rules: you have to do what's right for you and your important people.

If you decide to go down a treatment route, medication, therapy and other options such as exercise and coaching can be helpful – we cover these in the following chapter. Medication and therapy are incredibly effective for the majority (not 100 per cent) of adults with ADHD. While these won't cure your ADHD, research shows that this combination is probably more effective than the treatments for any other known psychiatric condition.

SUMMARY

If you are one of the few people who has accessed an adult ADHD diagnosis, you will know how difficult it is to jump through those hoops. The process itself discriminates against the very traits of our disorder, requiring skills in organising, planning, form-filling, dealing with uncertainty, avoiding impostor syndrome, metacognition and many others. Unless you are part of a random screening programme, there is a 'bias' in formally diagnosed people for those with above-average coping skills, intelligence, creativity, privilege or just luck. This CAN make it appear that everyone with ADHD has a set of skills because of the disorder when, in fact, the flawed system has failed many people who aren't lucky enough to navigate that nightmare.

This is a bit like putting an ADHD assessment clinic at the top of Mount Everest and then being wildly surprised that everyone diagnosed with ADHD appears to be an expert in mountain climbing. It must be a biological advantage. This is survivor bias and it is very seductive to believe it.

That doesn't mean it is easy for us though. It just means we are the lucky ones. And what do we get for this extraordinary luck? The next chapter looks at the minefield that involves deciding on which treatment and support is right for you!

CHAPTER 7

ADHD treatment

Adult ADHD is a treatable disorder for most people who have it. Treating and supporting adults with ADHD has clear benefits for all of society too.[37] A study from Israel found that for every dollar spent on ADHD treatment, over seven dollars were gained in lost revenue.[38] With this in mind, it just makes sense to support adults with ADHD.

In our experience, there are several stages in the journey of adults who are becoming aware that they have ADHD (although the stages aren't obligatory). These are undiagnosed, diagnosed, diagnosed and treated, and finally diagnosed and *managed*.

The difference between these last two stages may seem slight, but there is a world of difference between receiving treatment and receiving treatment *and* support that means you can more healthily succeed in life on a day-to-day basis. Undiagnosed and unsupported adults with ADHD have been calculated to have an 'economic burden' of around €20,000 per year (based on a study comparing adults to any non-ADHD siblings).[39] This figure seems largely due

ADHD UNPACKED

to factors such as reduced employment, increased sickness leave, reduced productivity, more accidents and more healthcare costs (this doesn't apply to everyone, though – this is on average). We think the moral and ethical value in ensuring that ADHD is properly treated and managed is reason enough, but it makes economic sense too!

We have talked a lot about the developmental brain differences that lead to ADHD and that it is usually treated with medicines. It might be a mistake that in many countries ADHD is grouped together with other mental health conditions and is therefore diagnosed and treated by experts in the field of psychiatry (and sometimes psychology). In countries such as Germany, ADHD is often treated as a neurological condition (such as epilepsy). While many people are sceptical of whether and how ADHD should be treated, especially in terms of medication, there is probably no other psychiatric condition or 'disorder' that responds better to medication than ADHD. Medication isn't the *only* treatment for ADHD, but in many countries it is the cornerstone of treatment.

If you are the type of person (like Alex) who actually reads the ridiculously long-winded information sheets that come with medication, printed using text so small you need a magnifying glass, you might accidentally find a really interesting sentence in the ADHD medication leaflet. This sentence will probably say something like, 'This medication is not intended to be used alone in treating ADHD; it must be combined with other therapeutic approaches.' Medication can be effective for most people, *but it should not be used alone!*

ADHD TREATMENT

Healthcare systems across the globe tend to treat ADHD with a similar combination of medication, talking therapies and psychoeducation (which is the structured delivery of education about a health condition to a patient). Some countries, such as Japan and Sweden, tend to avoid the use of medication and instead focus on education and therapy. The 'Updated European Consensus Statement on diagnosis and treatment of adult ADHD' even includes this statement: 'The treatment of adults with ADHD should follow a multimodal and multidisciplinary approach, which includes psychoeducation, pharmacotherapy, cognitive behavioural therapy (CBT) and coaching for ADHD.'[40]

If you have been diagnosed with ADHD, how many of these treatment approaches have you received? We will take a rough guess at one, maybe two. Possibly none. We are not naïve, and we know that these treatments are not permanent cures, nor will they solve all of the problems faced by adults with ADHD. However, in various forms, they can help us to concentrate and be more productive in achieving tasks and goals, and also help related issues such as anxiety.

Adults in the UK (and in most countries) who have been diagnosed with ADHD are usually offered medication. Some people choose not to take medication, and many find that medication doesn't work or causes intolerable side-effects. Others have additional conditions so the medication isn't suitable for them. These groups are often offered some talking therapies, such as cognitive behavioural therapy (CBT).

And that's it.

To compound this frankly pathetically inadequate level of support, talking therapies such as CBT are unlikely to work effectively in most adults with ADHD unless these are provided by a therapist with specific ADHD expertise (ADHD-informed therapy). Before we talk about this and what could be done about it, we want to briefly explain the different treatments for ADHD and how they are thought to work in our brains.

Medication

All ADHD medications work by increasing the levels of brain chemicals called neurotransmitters, such as dopamine, although other neurotransmitters are available. These brain chemicals appear to have decreased activity in the brains of people with ADHD. It is interesting that we don't seem to have *less* dopamine, rather the ability of dopamine to do its job is *worse*. Despite this, increasing the levels of these brain chemicals often reduces many of the core symptoms of ADHD, which are thought to be due in part to these brain chemicals not working properly.

In most countries, there are four different medications typically licensed and offered to adults with ADHD (there is a fifth licensed only for children called guanfacine). Three of these medications are known as stimulants. Although the word 'stimulant' isn't exactly a scientific term, these medicines generally target the brain to increase alertness, attention and energy. The other medication (called atomoxetine) is a 'non-stimulant' and a drug that was formerly used to treat depression but was also found to improve ADHD symptoms

ADHD TREATMENT

in some people (we are also unsure why this isn't called a stimulant too). In some countries, stimulant medications aren't legally available, which can limit treatment options.

There are slight differences in how the three stimulant and one non-stimulant medications are thought to work in the brain. Briefly, they all affect levels of neurotransmitters:

Stimulant medications

- Methylphenidate (such as Ritalin) increases the levels of dopamine and noradrenaline.

- Dexamphetamine (such as Dexedrine) increases the levels of dopamine, noradrenaline and serotonin.

- Lisdexamphetamine (such as Elvanse) increases the levels of dopamine, noradrenaline and serotonin.

Non-stimulant medication

- Atomoxetine (such as Straterra) is said to increase levels of noradrenaline only, but is increasingly thought to lead to an increase of dopamine as well.[41]

Collectively, these four drugs are effective in an impressive-sounding 80 per cent of adults with ADHD. If you look more closely at what 'effective' means, however, this varies from person to person. For some people, medication can make everyday tasks a little bit easier (still pretty useful). In others, it can have a genuinely profound impact on most aspects of day-to-day function.

Many people have said to us, 'Oh my God, this is how other people's brains work?' when they first get treatment for ADHD, whereas others say they felt a small effect that was hard to measure. Like all ADHD treatments, medication isn't a cure. We use the word 'cure' very tentatively, because some people in the ADHD community, particularly those who see their ADHD as a strength, don't like the idea of ADHD being something that should be cured. We think that view should be absolutely respected. A more inclusive alternative phrasing might be that medication won't entirely remove the more damaging personal symptoms of ADHD in anyone who takes it.

Like all medications, there are often side effects. These can vary but some common examples include a dry mouth, a loss of appetite and headaches, but you can find a lot more by reading the package insert that comes with your ADHD medication. There are bigger concerns around side effects to stimulant medication, such as suspected heart and blood vessel (cardiovascular) issues (with lisdexamphetamine in particular). These fears seem to be a bit unfounded, and a 2022 study showed that despite people with ADHD facing higher levels of heart disease (possibly for lifestyle or environmental reasons), this risk wasn't increased by the use of stimulant medication (or non-stimulants, for that matter).[42]

Some weaker studies appear to have found a side effect relating to blood pressure in some people, but in 2019 (partly due to this), UK NICE guidelines amended the recommendation on assessment for people starting medication for ADHD. The guidelines now indicate that a heart rhythm scan (called an ECG or echocardiogram) is NOT needed before starting

ADHD TREATMENT

the stimulants atomoxetine or guanfacine if that person's cardiovascular history and examination are normal and they aren't on a medicine that increases their cardiovascular risk.[43] Some doctors in the UK and in many other countries still request an annual ECG and blood test profile.

Because of these side effects (and because we all respond differently), a careful process of 'titration' is used by the mental health team. During titration, medication dosages are increased over several weeks, while symptoms and side effects are recorded (or should be). This usually leads to a safer and more effective dosage level to be reached on an individual patient basis.

Sometimes, the effects of these medications are subtle. As people with ADHD can be less able to identify if their symptoms have changed, it can help to have someone external to assess any impact. When James finished titration, for example, he told his psychiatrist that the medication had done 'fuck all', when in fact every single symptom had improved according to a chart he had to fill in.

It isn't uncommon and is perfectly sensible for adults with ADHD to be hesitant when offered medicine to treat the disorder. Every single medication for any condition has some kind of risk associated with it, and it is natural to be medication-hesitant or even to reject a medication approach completely. Having said that, this reticence sometimes stems from unreliable information from the internet or media. It can even come from a lack of understanding of what ADHD medication actually does, or from the stigma around ADHD medication that lingers from the '1980s Ritalin children' perception of 'zombie people' wandering around without their former personality. Choosing to accept medication is always a personal decision and one that we think should be made with full knowledge of both the benefits and potential side effects.

What about coffee and caffeine?

Caffeine levels vary wildly from one coffee to another, and this might be one of the reasons why it has stopped being used as a second-line treatment for ADHD (it used to be). Some researchers think that caffeine has been mistakenly excluded from ADHD medication lists in adults and could be useful in the treatment of mild/moderate adult ADHD. This is partly because caffeine is the ONLY psychoactive drug in the world that isn't really regulated by any culture and, more importantly, because a number of systematic reviews and meta-analyses (including this one from 2022[44]) found that caffeine use can promote alertness, attention and other elements. This may be because caffeine effectively blocks a chemical called adenosine, which itself stops our old friend dopamine from working. So, adenosine blocks dopamine, but caffeine blocks adenosine from blocking dopamine. To put it another way, more caffeine equals more dopamine activity. Before you rush off to the coffee shop for an ADHD cure, the studies are quite weak, so read into this as you will.

Therapy and coaching

If ADHD medication isn't appropriate or is poorly tolerated – or if someone falls into the 20 per cent of people for whom it isn't effective (or they simply make the personal decision not to take medication) – the next option is usually a talking therapy such as cognitive behavioural therapy (CBT). Sometimes, CBT is offered in addition to medication if medication alone hasn't improved symptoms in more than one area of life. This isn't common in our experience and really makes a mockery of that statement that 'medication should be combined with other therapeutic approaches'.

CBT focuses on challenging and changing unhelpful thoughts, attitudes, feelings and behaviours, with a therapist assisting to encourage healthy coping strategies that target specific problems. In people with ADHD, CBT aims to change the thoughts and behaviours that reinforce the harmful effects of ADHD, but it also helps people to cope with emotions, such as anxiety and depression, and improve self-esteem – all issues that are very common in ADHD.

So far, so good, right? There is also a huge amount of research into CBT and ADHD, and much of it suggests that CBT can be effective for treating adults with ADHD, especially when it is combined with ADHD medication. It is understandable why it is generally the 'second line' of treatment for many adults with ADHD. Look deeper though, and the evidence for use of CBT in ADHD starts to crumble a little.

The UK's NICE[45] and a review of evidence by the Cochrane Group (probably the world's most trusted source of testing the quality of clinical research studies[46]) both agree that there is 'low-quality evidence' that CBT may be beneficial for treating adults with ADHD in the short term. The

ADHD UNPACKED

evidence is largely classed as 'low quality' due to inconsistent or inaccurate results in various clinical trials.

Why is this important? The *British Medical Journal* summed it up well in an article that noted, 'Basing treatment decisions or clinical guidelines on low-quality evidence means that the true effects of a treatment or clinical decision might differ considerably from best estimates.'[47] We had to read that a few times to make sense of it. In other words, it might work, but it might not. If you had heart disease and your doctor offered you medication saying, 'This might work, or not, we don't really know,' we are sure you'd feel a touch let down by your healthcare system.

Beyond CBT, there are other talking therapies with *some* evidence of effectiveness. These techniques, which all work in different ways, include:

- **Dialectical Behavioural Therapy (DBT):** DBT should really be thought of as a type of CBT that focuses on building skills for regulating emotions, improving interpersonal relationships, and tolerating distress. DBT is more commonly used for personality disorders at the moment, but there is increasing interest in using it for ADHD support.

- **Eye Movement Desensitisation and Reprocessing (EMDR):** EMDR helps to reprocess traumatic memories so these are no longer distressing.

- **Assisted Relaxation Therapy (ART):** ART aims to help people reduce their stress, anxiety and tension

ADHD TREATMENT

through relaxation techniques guided and supported by a trained therapist or practitioner.

The evidence for these therapies working in ADHD is limited or in the early stages of being properly investigated.

Alongside talking therapy sits coaching. Coaching isn't a treatment, and a coach is not a therapist. Coaching is supposed to be (according to the European Union who wrote the elegantly titled Professional Charter for Coaching, Mentoring and Supervision of Coaches, Mentors and Supervisors[48]), 'A professional relationship in which a coach works with an individual or a group to help them achieve specific personal or professional goals.'

ADHD coaching is a specialised form of coaching aimed at helping people better manage their symptoms, improve their daily functioning and achieve their goals. As both Alex and James coach people with ADHD, we have to acknowledge a bias here, but there is growing evidence that coaching is an effective tool in managing the day-to-day challenges of living with ADHD. *If* you get a good coach.

Lifestyle changes

For the huge swathes of adults who have to wait for years to get assessed for ADHD, or for whom current therapies are ineffective, the search for alternatives can be a desperate one. Some lifestyle changes might help with managing ADHD symptoms and we think some of these are definitely worth exploring.

There is a lot of evidence that exercise can be useful in managing ADHD symptoms, with some studies suggesting that even a single bout of exercise is able to immediately improve ADHD symptoms (for a short while). However, there is little, if any, robust evidence on which types of exercise might work best and what the longer-term effects are. It might not matter exactly which kind of exercise you do, because there is pretty solid evidence that exercise can increase the activity of the brain chemicals such as dopamine that are increased by stimulant medication.

It is probably no surprise then, that when you look at research on exercise and ADHD in children, there is clear evidence to show that exercise improves inattention. While this is yet another example of 'more research needed', physical activity is good for general health and something to be encouraged. A challenge that adults with ADHD face is that evidence shows their symptoms can include being less likely to be physically active and facing more barriers to accessing physical activity. Although we might be more likely to impulsively join a gym (James paid upfront for a year's gym membership, not once but twice, and in both cases, only went once!), are we as likely to actually use the gym? Probably not!

As we will cover in Chapter 15, sleep issues and ADHD are very often linked. It has been suggested that a lack of sleep is more damaging to our daily function than *all* our ADHD symptoms combined, so improving sleep quality will likely help to manage ADHD symptoms.[49] It is in its early stages, but it is possible that morning light therapy, melatonin and even weighted blankets might be able to help improve sleep in ADHD adults, and therefore also help to manage symptoms. We would also recommend reducing the light in your bedroom as much as possible, trying to keep your bedroom cooler than the rest of your rooms, avoiding alcohol, caffeine and cigarettes, and trying to go to sleep (and wake up) at the same time every day, even at weekends. None of those suggestions are simple for anybody, least of all those of us with ADHD, but they are worth giving a go.

In terms of diet and nutritional changes, despite a lot of confident advice from many places about ADHD, there isn't a lot of evidence supporting any nutritional change to improve ADHD symptoms. To put that simply, ADHD is unlikely to be helped by changing your diet unless you have a very specific deficiency (such as a measurable iron deficiency) or a wildly unhealthy relationship with food. For most of us, this isn't going to be beneficial, but selling expensive dietary products is a very well-established money-making model.

Supplements and alternative therapies

With trust in pharmaceutical companies ranging between 31 per cent and 80 per cent[50] across different countries, it is easy to understand how many people prefer to turn to 'natural' supplements to either keep healthy or treat ailments.

What many people don't realise is that many common pharmaceutical drugs come from plants and other natural sources, and many of the vitamin supplements that people take are made synthetically. There isn't clear evidence for what we mean by 'natural' or whether there is a measurable difference in biological health. It often just feels right.

While there is some evidence that some supplements really can help with maintaining health in general, any dietary intervention should be done with the same level of care as starting a course of pharmaceutical medicines because, and we can't stress this enough, everything is a chemical whether it is natural or synthetic. Because the liver, the body's factory for breaking down and removing chemicals, does this with many of the things we ingest, taking supplements can interfere with how some medicines work (even some fruits such as grapefruit can affect this!). FYI: neither of us are 'in the pocket' of Big Pharma. We wish we were, as neither of us is very rich and James has more ADHD tax debt than most small countries – listen to episode 32 (The ADHD Tax) of our *The ADHD Adults Podcast* at https://podcasts.apple.com/us/podcast/episode-32-the-adhd-tax/id1591127163?i=1000566191520 if you want to learn more!

Because of the marked increase of people realising they may have ADHD, companies selling supplements are increasingly selling products online to 'treat' ADHD with little or no evidence or regulation to hold them to account for their claims. This is another potential gold mine for those peddling snake oil. Or fish oil, for that matter.

The evidence in favour of a general positive effect of using natural supplements to help with ADHD symptoms is weak. Individually, using supplements such as fish oils, magnesium, vitamin D and iron *may* help with ADHD symptoms, but this is usually in people who already have a deficiency in those nutrients and are therefore just getting them to the correct levels in the body. The supplement with the most evidence for helping to manage ADHD symptoms is probably omega-3 (sometimes, studies specifically use fish oil), but the evidence is mixed, finding that it either helps or does nothing, so it is hard to draw clear conclusions. It is likely that eating a healthy, nutrient-dense diet is a better way of maintaining these nutrient levels than any single thing UNLESS your doctor identifies a specific medical deficiency. There can also be negative effects of making dietary changes without consulting your ADHD specialist, such as the build-up of toxins or effects on ADHD medication.

One of the more interesting non-pharmaceutical 'sort of dietary' approaches gathering interest is functional or 'magic' mushrooms helping with ADHD symptoms. Although microdosing magic mushrooms has some weak evidence to support this claim, this usually comes from 'self-reports'. These kinds of studies are less reliable because self-reports often (not always) reflect the placebo effect or a short-term response that goes away after a few weeks. Many people are also using lion's mane (a medicinal mushroom) for ADHD thanks to the internet saying it helps with ADHD symptoms such as focus. Currently, there is zero scientific evidence to support this.

We often get accused of not supporting these alternative remedies out of a sort of prohibitionist mindset. This is ironic, as we have been advocates for the research into illegal medications and ADHD for many years. As soon as there is relatively believable evidence, we will shout it from the rooftops.

It isn't all bad news delivered by two bitter ex-academics, however. There may be no clear positive dietary interventions, but there *is* evidence that mindfulness can help to manage some ADHD symptoms and associated issues such as anxiety.[51] In our experience, when you mention mindfulness to most adults with ADHD, you will get an eye-roll. The thought of even trying to sit still and quieten one's mind seems ludicrous, but mindfulness comes in many forms and for some, it can help. Alex has practised ADHD-friendly mindfulness for decades, including one-minute breathing exercises, meditating while doing other enjoyable activities and mindfulness in interesting or noisy environments.

You can sometimes find dubious papers encouraging alternative approaches, including homeopathy, acupuncture or so-called emotional freedom techniques (EFT) such as tapping, in treating ADHD. Again, this research is often poorly designed or biased. There are no proper clinical trials demonstrating evidence for any of these. While they are mostly not harmful to try, they tend to be grouped as a belief system of pseudoscience that is unlikely to be of measurable benefit outside an occasional placebo effect. The American National Center for Complementary and Integrative Health says that homeopathy hasn't been shown to be helpful for ADHD or anxiety. It is also important to note that no homeopathic products are approved by the Food and Drug Administration (FDA).[52]

With all these approaches, it is important to say that an absence of evidence isn't the same as evidence of an absence (a cool sentence to learn for parties). Sometimes,

ADHD TREATMENT

we are just so far behind with good research that we don't yet know if something works.

So, how should ADHD be treated?

This is something we have given a great deal of thought. What is currently offered to people once they are diagnosed with ADHD is clearly not sufficient, but what should post-diagnostic care look like? We feel that adults with ADHD should be offered the following once they receive a diagnosis:

- medication (if they want it)
- therapy (if they need it, which they usually do)
- ADHD-informed coaching (of course we think that)
- structured and evidence-based psychoeducation
- sleep training (if they need it)
- support with ANY coexisting condition.

We would also stress the importance of the relationship with any therapist or coach as fundamental, combined with an ADHD-informed conversation, which is often referring to the need for individualistic or person-centred talking therapy.

We are working hard trying to advocate to make this a reality. We know there are economic, political and cultural barriers, but as public awareness and (hopefully) political support increase, we live in hope that one day treating ADHD properly will be given the importance it clearly requires.

SUMMARY

ADHD is a disorder with multiple treatment options and can be treated and managed with appropriate support. With the various treatment options for ADHD, there should be a post-diagnostic support package available for every adult with ADHD to help them manage their symptoms on a day-to-day basis. This support isn't always made available to everyone, even though there is strong evidence that treating ADHD leads to better outcomes for not just people with ADHD, but society as a whole. Trying to get meaningful evidence for supplements, lifestyle changes or new suggestions on the internet is fraught with difficulty.

There is a lot of research out there, but much of it has usually been done on a budget or with some kind of bias in mind. This is often described by the teams trying to compare the science with a meta-analysis of the data as 'garbage in, garbage out' (or GIGO). Regardless of your opinion on treatment or your access to treatment in the first place, some or all of the core challenges of attentional issues, hyperactivity and impulsivity are going to be present and probably disruptive. We will discuss attention in the next chapter, followed by a combined chapter on hyperactivity and impulsivity, before we move on to the ways in which ADHD affects us personally and professionally.

CHAPTER 8

Pay attention!

By this point, some of you may have drifted away more than once, possibly thinking about anything other than adult ADHD. That is both ironic, and also probably not your fault. ADHD is literally a disorder that includes *not being able to pay attention to what we want to pay attention* to, and this has a profound impact on many people.

That second part of that description of inattention is often wildly misunderstood. This is key to another of those misconceptions that those of us with ADHD 'don't want' to pay attention to something or someone. Obviously, that can be partly true sometimes (as it would be for anyone), but very often we desperately, eagerly, *want* to pay attention to a task that we absolutely know is a priority. However, the parts of our brain that manage what we pay attention to decide that they will instead direct our attention towards something else, such as playing a game on our phone (James) or learning all the kings and queens of England in order (Alex). As inattention is usually a core issue with ADHD, it helps to first discuss what attention is, and how it is usually controlled by the brain.

What do we mean by 'attention'?

Attention is surprisingly difficult to define, with opinions from psychologists helpfully ranging from 'Everyone knows what attention is' to 'No one knows what attention is'. Despite these insightful psychological opinions, we would generally define attention as 'the ability to focus on specific information or tasks while tuning out other details or thoughts'. The word 'ability' does a lot of the heavy lifting in this definition, but it immediately raises a bit of red flag for what ADHD is.

Do we have the ability to pay attention to things we want to? Yes, we have that ability. Of course, we do (mostly). Do we consistently apply this ability to pay attention to things we want to? That's a big no.

What this shows us is that ADHD is often a *performance* issue, not an *ability* issue – we are usually consistently *inconsistent* when it comes to attention.

Abilities vary from person to person, and this doesn't mean we all have the ability to pay attention all of the time. For example, we can't all run 100 metres in 9.58 seconds like Usain Bolt. He was able to run 100 metres at that speed. Those of us without mobility challenges also have the ability to successfully run 100 metres, but in a time that is much slower than Bolt's. But, and this is a big but: *Bolt only ran the 100 metres at this speed once.* This means that although he had the *ability* to do it, he couldn't perform at that level consistently. If he did that every hour, he would face a lot of physical (and probably emotional) damage very quickly.

PAY ATTENTION!

Almost any ability exists in ranges, and the performance is what enables us to apply our ability to do things consistently (or well). The ability to pay attention to thoughts, tasks or people isn't much different. Technically, while we *can* do it sometimes (we have the ability), we might be more easily distracted and often we can't do it consistently. Performance — not ability. Even if you can run a kilometre, you can't usually do it one hundred times in a row and you can't do it as fast as Usain Bolt. You have to choose what and when to do these things and to try and figure out how much that will cost physically and emotionally.

Types of attention

As far as attention is concerned, there are technically thought to be five different types, which we will now discuss in the first of a series of boring lists.

1. *Focused attention*: Or 'Look, a squirrel!' This is when we are paying attention to a single task or activity without being distracted by what is going on around us. An example of this might be the ability to revise for an exam while the television is on.

2. *Sustained attention*: Or 'watching *The Godfathe*r'. This is when we hold attention on a single task that takes some time. This might occur when you get lost in a good book or watch a long film.

3. *Selective attention*: Or 'the divorce defence'. This is when we can block out a number of things happening around us to focus on just one thing. An

example of this is focusing on one person's voice in a room full of conversations or when the television is on.

4. *Divided attention*: Or 'the taxi driver'. This is multitasking or focusing on two or more things at the same time (such as talking to your customer in the taxi and complaining about the state of politics). People often say that multitasking is difficult for people (and men especially), but most people can do it (albeit with differing levels of success and depending on the parts of the brain needed to do the different tasks). Holding a conversation while driving is a good example: easy when you have been driving for years, but not so easy when you are seventeen and still learning what the left-hand pedal does. This has been called the highest level of attention.

5. *Alternating Attention*: Or 'The ADHD one, let's be honest'. This is switching your focus from one activity to another, such as stopping typing an email to answer your phone. Or writing a book and also constantly checking the internet, for example.

Unsurprisingly, people with inattentive-type or combined-type ADHD will, by definition, find challenges in some or even all of these forms of attention. Three of these (namely sustained attention, selective attention and alternating attention) are generally more difficult for people with ADHD. Focused attention, on just one task, is an issue for many people, especially as there are distractions everywhere. But the odd thing about ADHD is that we can sometimes 'hyperfocus'.

Hyperfocus (or hyperfixation)

Hyperfocus has been defined as 'locking on' to a task, even if the task isn't necessarily an objective priority or something that is usually of interest to that person. It is an intense state of concentration that has even been compared to a 'hypnotic spell'. Although this is probably familiar to many people with ADHD, there is no clear scientific definition of hyperfocus, and some refer to it as a 'hyperfixation'.

When someone is engaged in hyperfocus, there is usually a big drop in our perception of what's going on around us, and even what is going on inside our body and mind. Examples of hyperfocus include becoming so engrossed in a video game that you don't even hear the phone ring or hear someone calling your name. You might also not even notice you are hungry or thirsty.

Although hyperfocus isn't unique to ADHD and is also frequently seen in non-ADHD adults, people with more ADHD symptoms generally report higher levels of, and more frequent, episodes of hyperfocus. Research has shown that a big difference between people with and without ADHD is that hyperfocus is less likely to occur in educational and social situations if you have ADHD (which seems unfair). This means hyperfocus is possibly not as useful for adults with ADHD as it is for other people in a school or college setting.

Sadly, we can't easily choose what we hyperfocus on, or it would legitimately be a superpower. Normally, our brain will engage us in in hyperfocus if a task is particularly rewarding. If you are fortunate enough to be able to hyperfocus on

ADHD UNPACKED

your work or hobbies, it can feel like a superpower! But if Superman couldn't control when his laser vision came on, it wouldn't be much of a superpower, would it? Think of the poor people of Metropolis. Some people have managed to build a career based on their hyperfocus, and legitimately consider this to be a superpower. We would agree for that one individual, but this isn't a common or consistent experience among most adults with ADHD.

Evidence suggests that the highest level of attention, so-called multitasking or 'divided attention', may be less of a problem for many people with ADHD, but remember that we are all different and this could also be an issue for individuals. Some of us can multitask away (and even prefer to work in that way), while others need to remove all distractions, finding it impossible to have more than one thing to focus on and be successful at it. We sometimes joke that ADHD people split into 'need the radio on to work' and 'can't have the radio on to work'.

Task switching

Most people know that many adults with ADHD have issues with focusing our attention (it *is* in the name). But there can also be a problem with changing what we are paying attention to. This process of switching our attention from one task to another (and possibly back again) is called 'task switching' for obvious reasons. Most brains can handle working on two simple jobs at once by switching focus from one to the other when needed (such as listening to an amateurish podcast while doing the washing up). But trying to focus on two (or more) complex tasks at the same time is a lot more challenging (such as listening to instructions on how to get somewhere at the same time as changing a tyre on your car). This is difficult for everyone, especially if the aim is to do them both well and/or quickly, but ADHD adults seem to struggle more than average, both in switching tasks in the first place and in staying on task, even when we want to remain focused.

Unfortunately, being able to switch attention from one task to another is fundamentally important in life, and though switching attention between tasks can feel good (if the alternative task is pleasant or at least not dead boring), this has an impact on the brain. Task switches require mental control, effort and time, all of which use up some of the brain's bandwidth.

Most task switching is unconscious (or subconscious, if you prefer). This means that we don't have to deliberately plan it by actively thinking about it. As an example, if your phone starts ringing while you are writing a (fascinating ADHD) book, you don't usually have to consciously say to yourself, 'I'll stop writing this book now and will answer the phone instead.' Usually, the ringing phone can trigger our brain to stop reading and switch to the other task subconsciously. We just seem to do it. Or we don't. Because task switching can be harder with ADHD because our brains are generally less able to mentally prepare for switching tasks. Even when we receive a cue to change tasks (such as a phone call), we can struggle to stop doing the first one in order to start doing the second. A lack of cognitive flexibility, distractibility, poor working memory and other core ADHD issues make this switch really difficult at times.

There are four things the brain needs to do to allow us to switch tasks; **STOP** the first task, **SWITCH** focus to the second task, **START** the second task and finally **MAINTAIN** focus on the second task (without drifting back to the first ... or doing something else...). All of these steps require the executive functions that adults with ADHD usually don't have a great deal of. This isn't impossible, but it is very often difficult.

In everyday life, we *have to* 'task switch' a lot. Life is a series of task switches, separated by periods of staring into the abyss and eating biscuits (also a task). Here is an (in no way typical or relatable) scenario to illustrate this:

A very kind and patient editor is sitting at her computer, attempting to chase up the two authors of an adult ADHD book who are several months behind schedule and not answering their emails. The phone rings, and she answers. It is her boss, demanding a printed copy of what has been written so far before her boss kills the project and possibly the two hapless authors. The very kind and patient editor searches her computer, finds the document containing what has been submitted so far, clicks 'Print', gets up from her desk and goes to the printer (chatting to Janet on the way, who has had to take her dog to the vet as it ate an entire chicken leg and required surgery). She collects the pages from the printer and carries it to her boss's office.

This sequence of more than ten tasks requires multiple 'task switches', each time applying those four steps of *stopping*, *switching*, *starting* and *focusing*. That is a lot of executive functioning. Now if this kind and patient editor

PAY ATTENTION!

had ADHD, chances are that even though some of the tasks had prompts, such as the phone call and Janet saying, 'Hi', at some point in this seemingly simple, multi-step process, there is likely to be a moment when things grind to a halt as the brain just says, 'No!' We never know which task is going to overload the system, even tasks we have done before with no problem. Even tasks we usually enjoy.

As it often does with ADHD, all this talk of attention comes back to the brain itself. Why is attention a problem at all? Surely with our super-evolved brains being so incredible, having what is effectively unlimited storage capacity, a simple thing like attention should be an open goal? While the human brain truly *is* amazing, with a massive memory capacity, it *does not* have unlimited 'bandwidth' to take in or process information, just like a smartphone or computer. If your laptop has ever frozen even if it still has memory available, or you have ever had to restart your phone to get its apps to work properly, then you understand this problem. This issue is often because the processor has become overwhelmed despite plenty of room for memory left on the hard drive.

When it comes to what the brain can and will process, there is simply too much information coming into the brain for us to handle. Our brain has to deal with a metaphorical (hopefully) tidal wave of information every second, bombarding it from both inside and outside our body. If you just consider sight, each eye alone delivers around 1 Mb of data *every second* to the brain.[53] When you add this to all the other information flung haphazardly towards our brains, it requires a powerful system to 'select' which information from this torrent of data to focus on. This could be information about

143

what is going on around you, or information your thoughts are generating for themselves.

Our attention is therefore split between those things happening around us in our environment and the biological stuff going on inside us (such as how fast our heart is beating, or if we are dehydrated). We also have to pay attention to what goes on in our thoughts. In any case, our 'bandwidth' is limited, so our brain must select to which information it allocates our attention. And it isn't always perfect at this.

Imagine, if you can, sitting in an office environment, which can (not always) be torturous for people with ADHD. You have an important report to write with a looming deadline, but your email inbox keeps popping up with notifications. On top of that, your mobile phone beeps each time someone messages you, and the accountancy department, in the cubicle next to you, is talking loudly about ... erm ... numbers? For most people, staying focused on the report (the important thing) isn't too much of a problem as they have a brain that can (to some extent) filter out the other distractions (apart from the accountants – some things are universally distracting).

Everyone can get distracted, but this 'filtering' of information is usually more difficult for people with ADHD (or at least the ones who have issues with inattention, which is more than 90 per cent of us). This is because of those differences in our brains, especially in the parts that do the filtering of those distractions and select or switch what we pay attention to. In the human brain, several areas have evolved to take this job on.

PAY ATTENTION!

The first area is a sort of central controller in the brain. Like a doctor's receptionist but not as terrifying. This controller has to make sense of all the information coming in, while there are multiple tasks simultaneously requiring our attention, and make 'decisions' about which elements to engage with and which to ignore. This control centre for attention in the brain is called the pre-frontal cortex, which essentially means 'the very front of the front bit of the outside of the brain' (we like how silly brain names are). This alternative description hopefully gives you an idea of where the pre-frontal cortex is – behind your forehead, mostly on the right-hand side.

The pre-frontal cortex will be mentioned a few times in this chapter, as it is involved in almost all aspects of ADHD symptoms, so we will call it the PFC from now on to save ink. Importantly, the PFC doesn't work alone. In fact, almost no area of your brain works in isolation. As attention is a process required for all your thoughts, movements and bodily functions that involve different areas of the brain, everything the brain does happens in coordination with those networks of connected brain areas that we talked a lot about in Chapter 3. These areas of the brain work together like members of a team to get stuff done. With ADHD, however, they don't talk to each other in the same way and tend to be 3–0 down at half-time.

One of the jobs of the PFC is to coordinate the conscious 'decisions' about what we pay attention to, such as writing a report, listening to those accountants or remembering that we have shortened pre-frontal cortex to PFC. It also coordinates the so-called unconscious (or subconscious) 'decisions', such as thinking about how the report will prob-ably get you an indifferent response from your boss.

Calling these 'decisions' is a bit unhelpful as in many cases your brain is making the decision for you, so it doesn't feel much like a choice. Rather, the brain assesses information on its own and directs a response, such as focusing on the report. And in ADHD, the PFC, along with its teammates, is often not very good at directing this. This leads to issues with selecting what we pay attention to (and for how long). That, in a nutshell, is what inattentiveness is.

Distractions and attention

If you are indeed paying attention, you may have noticed the word 'distraction' or 'distracted' has popped up several times so far in this chapter. It isn't unfair to say that most adults with ADHD could be described as 'distractible'. But not always — and distractions come in many forms. This might include background noise in a restaurant, daydreaming about going on holiday next year, or something appearing in the window.

Modern life is full of distractions. Take a second now, put this book down and look around at your environment (but please, please remember to pick it back up again). What can you see that might be a distraction for you personally? We would imagine at least a mobile phone, possibly a window, even another person. On top of all that, there is also *you* (although you probably won't see yourself unless there is a mirror nearby).

PAY ATTENTION!

Hopefully, now you are picking the book back up, so we can tell you that all of these things can distract you from tasks you are trying to engage with. And there are many more things in everyday life that will act as distractions to take you away from anything you are trying to allocate your attention to. Some of these are 'tempting' ones. These are often more enjoyable or fun than the task at hand, such as watching Netflix or eating a cake. Some distractions can also include temptations, even if these aren't particularly fun, providing quick rewards (such as pointless and repetitive games on your phone).

Separate types of distraction, which are far less fun, are aversive distractions. These are less pleasant activities you also feel need to be done, such as tidying the kitchen or clearing out the garage. James has a saying for this: 'If you want somebody to clean your house, ask someone with ADHD to do a different job instead.' If we (or more accurately, our subconscious) are trying to allocate our attention to a task that we seem to find unrewarding in the short term, then even deep cleaning the oven is something our brain may direct us to do instead. Much of this is due to the need to feel reward, which we discuss a lot more in Chapter 10.

If your brain's reward centre finds a task or activity emotionally rewarding (in the relative short term), it will be easier to engage with it. If your brain's reward centre doesn't see where it will get a feeling of reward from, it is highly likely to seek out and direct you to engage in something that it finds rewarding instead, even if that thing is cleaning the house.

Unfortunately for those of us with ADHD, knowing intellectually that you will be rewarded one day is not the same as your subconscious brain centre feeling that the reward of this task right now is worth letting you do it (such as saving money or preparing for an important meeting in a week). We will often then be 'distracted' and do or think about something else instead. These distractions can be separated into 'external distractions' and 'internal distractions', which we will explore below.

External distractions

For most people, the word 'distraction' usually refers to external things that happen, such as a phone ringing. Much of the research into ADHD and distractibility has focused on these external distractions and, as a result, our understanding about distractibility comes from how our brains struggle to filter out external things. Partly because of this, external distractibility is considered to be a core diagnostic criterion for ADHD.

External things that you hear, see, smell or feel, which are unrelated to the task you are trying to pay attention to, are sometimes called 'task-irrelevant' distractions. These appear more likely to disrupt the ability to pay attention in people with ADHD than in people without it. Often, all we can do to try and control this is to limit the distractions around us. Sadly, this means phones often need to be put away! Alex makes sure his phone charger is not by his bed, for example. This also helps with getting to sleep.

Internal distractions

The *really* interesting stuff about distractibility occurs not outside the body, but inside our heads. It is difficult enough

PAY ATTENTION!

having to deal with the modern world where almost everything seems to be designed to distract us from what we are supposed to be doing (thanks, Angry Birds). In addition to so many social media platforms, mobile phone apps and interesting-looking dogs on the street, we also have myriad internal distractions that can take us away from tasks and activities that we genuinely do want to focus on (and sometimes don't).

Possibly the most intrusive of these is mind wandering.

Mind wandering occurs when someone's attention sort of drifts away from the task they are focused on in favour of a series of various thoughts or images, often for no obvious reason at all. This isn't just an 'ADHD thing' as it happens to everyone from time to time, possibly making up 50 per cent of most people's daily thinking time. Planned mind wandering, a bit like daydreaming, can be a useful thing for reflection and personal development. But have you ever been in the middle of a conversation (even if you really are trying to listen) when suddenly your thoughts take you somewhere else? This is the other type of mind wandering – spontaneous mind wandering – and that is well … not so great.

Spontaneous mind wandering happens without any conscious planning. During a task or unrelated thought, our minds can start to flit from thought to thought and stop us from 'being in the room', so to speak. This isn't just a quirky trait. It can interfere with everyday tasks where paying attention can be *really* important, such as listening to someone giving crucial instructions or driving a forklift truck, but it can also create an intense sense of shame and damage relationships and careers without healthy and open communication.

ADHD UNPACKED

This kind of mind wandering, as you have probably guessed, can explain many of the attention issues that adults with ADHD have. If all of a sudden, you are thinking about something completely unrelated to what you want to pay attention to, it can seem very clear that you weren't listening, and people can interpret this as a sign that you don't care about them or that project. This isn't the right interpretation, but it is understandable from a neurotypical point of view – and that often feels very painful to live with.

Again, the reason behind this mind wandering is our beautiful but slightly dysfunctional brain. In Chapter 3, we introduced a series of connected brain parts or 'networks'. One of these was the 'default mode network' (or DMN, which Alex calls the DeMoN network because it is the relaxation demon). The DMN is also sometimes called the 'daydreaming network' and is the reason behind the mind wandering we have been describing. This network is active when we are fully awake but not really doing anything practical, in that kind of daydreaming or reflective state.

The interesting ADHD aspect is what happens when we go from being restful to trying to perform tasks. When this happens, another brain network, called the 'task positive network' (TPN), switches off the daydreaming parts of the brain. Sorry for all the complicated anatomical names – blame the neurophysiologists.

When you turn off the DMN and turn on the TPN, this enables you to drive that forklift truck without daydreaming and injuring someone. However, in ADHD this switch isn't fully functional, and the daydreaming parts of the brain don't seem to switch off properly. Despite being ready to get that task done, the daydreaming part of the brain is also still a bit ready to drag our focus away.

This can be a big problem if our brain is more likely to trigger daydreaming when we are meant to be focused on a crucial task requiring serious concentration. It is difficult to explain to a loved one that while they were sharing their heartfelt emotions with us, we were thinking about whether penguins have legs or just feet. The incidences of mind wandering and ADHD are so widespread that it has been suggested it might be a better predictor of ADHD-associated problems than the traditional ADHD symptoms of inattention and hyperactivity/impulsivity. Penguins do have legs. This lack of control over what we allocate our attention to leads to inattention.

Inattention

From a medical disorder perspective, issues with paying attention, at least in ADHD, are called 'inattentive' symptoms or traits. There are nine diagnostic symptoms of inattentiveness in the fifth edition of that Diagnostic Statistical Manual (DSMV), which you might remember from previous chapters is the thick and boring handbook of psychiatry. We have listed these symptoms in Chapter 6.

If you have ADHD, or suspect you have ADHD, or even if you are reading this book to better support a loved one (you rock!), it may be useful to look at these symptoms of inattention and reflect on whether they are something you recognise in yourself, or those you are trying to support.

You could also ask yourself, 'How often do they occur? Is this every now and then, or quite often every day?' If you have ADHD, the latter is more likely.

It is important to point out that *everybody* will occasionally recognise one or more of these symptoms in themselves or their colleagues. Who can honestly say that they have never put their keys down and been distracted from what they were doing? Who among us always likes tasks that require sustained mental effort?

However, to have a diagnosis of ADHD, you would need to experience at least five of these nine symptoms, pretty much all the time (it doesn't matter which five), and to the point where they have a negative impact on at least two areas of your life (such as work and home). These symptoms might range from not finding it easy to read simple instructions to putting your glasses down twenty times a day and instantly forgetting where you put them only to find them in the fridge (for example). It may be sending messages on your phone littered with typos, or a strange inability to empty the dishwasher or vacuum the stairs.

Remember, these aren't occasional, one-off problems. Actual ADHD feels like we can't do the seemingly simple tasks of everyday life almost constantly (even if we might do some of them sometimes or have done some of them the first time we tried). It is the daily impact of ADHD that people who don't have ADHD often struggle to comprehend. The simplest of tasks can feel difficult, or even impossible, to do; maddeningly, even if you have done them before.

These symptoms of inattentiveness can be infuriating, but de-weaponising ADHD through kindness and a sense of humour and perspective is a powerful approach to living more healthily and, honestly, inattentiveness can sometimes have hilarious consequences once you accept your ADHD isn't a choice or a weakness of character.

Can any adults with ADHD manage to put together a piece of flat-pack furniture correctly at the first attempt? Can we manage to sit through an entire three-and-a-half-hour film without a break? The answer is yes – some of us can. This is because we might share many of those symptoms and behaviours from the book, but how they manifest in each of us differs, based on personality and preferences.

We are *all* different, and if (like Alex) you quite enjoy putting together flat-pack furniture, it is perfectly feasible to get it right the first time (probably not every time, unless you have a good system). If you are more like James, you are likely to have accidentally built a series of Swedish-inspired modern art pieces in your house instead of a wardrobe. On the other hand, Alex can't watch any movie without at least twelve breaks, whereas James is quite happy to watch all of the *Twilight* films in a row (Alex made that last bit up). As we have mentioned, there is neurodiversity even within a neurodivergent population of people with ADHD. To adapt a common quote from the autistic community: when you have met one person with ADHD, you have met one person with ADHD.

SUMMARY

Most people with ADHD have attention problems. It is fundamental for the majority of us. There are no guaranteed answers for what you can do about it, but we have included some ideas that people find have helped them deal more peacefully with those challenges in Chapter 16.

More importantly, it is vital that we communicate with our loved ones that this isn't a lack of willpower or a personality weakness. Inattention also doesn't mean that we don't care about the topic or person – we often do. We don't choose to let our minds wander so much, and we don't control when it happens, but we do often feel that burning shame of coming 'back in the room' when someone says, 'So what do you think?'

Emotional acceptance of ADHD is a common theme whenever we talk about our developmental disorder. In the next chapter, we will discuss the other diagnostic side of ADHD that affects at least half of all ADHD adults: hyperactivity impulsivity.

CHAPTER 9

Sit still and don't interrupt!

It might seem an odd question, but do you say you have ADD or ADHD? What is your flavour? Most adults with ADHD have some level of hyperactivity and/or impulsivity, with only around 30 per cent of adults being purely 'inattentive'. Some people like to call this 'Attention Deficit Disorder' or ADD, as opposed to the more official and slightly longer (but equally useless) 'Hyperactive/Impulsive Presentation Attention Deficit Hyperactivity Disorder/ADHD'. ADD isn't a name medically used anymore, but it is still quite commonly heard in some parts of the world. So, what is hyperactivity, and its conjoined issue of impulsivity?

In simple terms, 'hyperactivity' is used to describe when a person can't easily stop the *urge* to move or think in general. 'Impulsivity' tends to describe when a person can't easily stop a specific thought or reaction. Combined, these issues form the other diagnostic list of ADHD symptoms in comparison with 'inattention' that we described in Chapter 8. Both hyperactivity and impulsivity are pretty similar and seem to stem from the brain not being able to stop (or inhibit) some movements, thoughts or actions. So, in both cases, there is a problem with the brakes of the brain.

In desperately dull and dry neurological terms, the 'inhibition' of thoughts and actions require a collection of brain processes in the same way that paying attention to a task does. These brain processes enable us to limit our impulsive thoughts and behaviours, control our reactions to events or emotions, and regulate our bodily movements. These are obviously quite important processes. The brains of people with ADHD can go fast but aren't so good at stopping themselves. The research also suggests that the processing speed of an average ADHD brain doesn't actually appear faster than the brain of anybody else.

Hyperactivity

Hyperactivity is a state of being abnormally active. From the outside, it is usually pretty easy to spot in someone with ADHD. Some of us may be always moving around (although we can mask this by sitting on our hands or just putting up with the internal screaming terror of 'not being allowed to move'). We may be the person sitting in a meeting constantly clicking our pen or swinging around in our seat. We may be the person waiting in the queue, swaying from side to side as we stand there. Some of us – take James, for example – physically can't take a phone call sitting down, instead prowling like a caged tiger as we talk on the phone. This is also the reason James can't sunbathe for more than three minutes and forty-seven seconds. It is infuriating.

SIT STILL AND DON'T INTERRUPT!

But this depiction of hyperactivity doesn't tell the whole picture. Plenty of people without ADHD prefer to walk while on the phone. ADHD hyperactivity is about the severity and how much you move compared to most people. Even more confusingly, for many adults with ADHD the hyperactivity *isn't* necessarily about excess physical movement, but is more about internal restlessness: an inability to switch off our thoughts or engage with relaxing activities. We will try to explain these types of hyperactivities, and impulsivity, in the rest of this chapter.

External hyperactivity

Move. Just move. The feeling of being physically hyperactive is difficult to describe. It is a little bit like having an internal itch that only gets scratched when you move – only the less you 'scratch' this internal itch, the more you feel that itch. Moving calms this feeling down a little and allows many people with ADHD to feel calmer inside. But that itch doesn't go away; for some of us, it is always there.

Another name for hyperactivity, one that was used in the past, is 'hyperkinetic movements' – this describes 'abnormal and involuntary movements,' which is also a pretty good description of external hyperactivity. Often, we find ourselves moving but weren't necessarily aware of 'the itch' to move. It can be quite a surprise to see ourselves on camera, for example.

This need to move is often why we appear hyperactive. Sitting still isn't just difficult but can be distressing. Internally, having to sit still when expected can feel like having a swarm of bees in your brain™ (Alex claims to have used this bee analogy first). Moving can feel like a beekeeper is smoking those bees, making them quieter and enabling a hyperactive person to feel less distressed. This isn't smoking them like a cigarette – the beekeepers are pumping smoke into their hives. We looked it up.

Movement in the human body is governed largely by a part of the brain called the 'motor cortex' (or the outside bit, if you prefer) at the top of the brain. In more than half of people with ADHD, this part of the brain doesn't communicate as well with other parts, such as the prefrontal cortex (which crops up in Chapter 11) and the oddly named 'basal ganglia' (which we mention again later in this chapter). The lack of proper communication between these brain areas (which are vital for regulating our movement) is partly to blame for external hyperactivity. Perhaps unsurprisingly, that famous ADHD neurotransmitter dopamine is also heavily involved in starting (and stopping) our body from moving around.

Another possible reason for hyperactivity is that the brain of someone with ADHD may be trying to compensate for a natural level of underactivity. If our brain has reduced activity of neurotransmitters such as dopamine, increasing our physical movement might be a trigger to increase their activity in the brain, possibly to improve focus and alertness. This might make some sense, such as jumping around in the cold to warm up our brain and get moving. The problem is that nobody knows for sure, and many of these explanations are based on educated guesses without a lot of solid evidence.

Internal hyperactivity

For many adults with ADHD (and disproportionately in women), hyperactivity isn't about excess movement. Even if we were hyperactive as children, as adults we can find that we have replaced that more obvious physical hyperactivity of childhood with a more internal feeling of restlessness. This is much harder to spot in people around you, but it often manifests itself as racing thoughts, not being able to 'switch off' and relax, and the feeling that you always have to be 'on the go'. It is *exhausting* to never be able to mentally switch off, to always have one or several thoughts competing in your brain and to not even be able to rest in the evening or at weekends as internally your brain plays the cruel trick of saying 'GET UP AND DO SOMETHING' but also 'I'M NOT GOING TO LET YOU DO ANYTHING'.

This is, frankly, really annoying. It is even possible that this internal restlessness makes the inattentive symptoms of ADHD more difficult to deal with because poor organisation and distractibility are also characteristics of internal restlessness. Alex coined the term 'domestic anxiety' for how difficult this restlessness can be – for example, the shame of not always being able to spend time quietly in the evenings with loved ones. This difficulty is where ADHD isn't just a problem with society. It can cause a lot of emotional stress, and many people (including us) observe this to be part of the reason for alcohol and substance use disorders.

Internal hyperactivity also commonly includes racing thoughts. A psychologist might describe these as 'a subjective acceleration and overproduction of thoughts', but an actual human might call them 'a stream of seemingly endless and unstoppable thoughts that happens every night when I switch the bedroom light off.' These thoughts can be overwhelming!

Have you ever had an earworm? This is a song that you just can't stop playing in your head. Well, racing thoughts are like that, but it isn't only music, and it is probably even less enjoyable. The thoughts can vary massively, focusing on a single topic or mixing multiple different lines of thought either at the same time or in a train of thinking that we can't just stop. These thoughts can be about anything, including issues at work, relationships or conversations we haven't yet had with Geoff at the office.

Because of the common link between ADHD and other conditions such as anxiety, these racing thoughts can also be particularly negative and self-destructive. Therapy to reframe them into a more positive mindset is genuinely important for many of us to emotionally accept our ADHD.

While racing thoughts are not just an ADHD thing (of course racing thoughts are found in the general population), they happen more often in adults with ADHD, as well as in some mental health conditions such as bipolar disorders, depression and insomnia. The cause of the racing thoughts can be difficult to identify, as these conditions often 'coexist' with ADHD. Racing thoughts aren't a new concept – they were described in 1858 as 'melancholia agitans' where patients 'cannot focus their thoughts; as soon as they form an idea, it disappears, and a completely different one quickly takes its place'.

SIT STILL AND DON'T INTERRUPT!

As if that wasn't enough, internal hyperactivity also appears to be connected to intrusive thoughts, which are subtly different to racing thoughts. Intrusive thoughts can be defined as repetitive, unwanted or unacceptable thoughts, images or impulses. These largely fall into two types: involuntary thoughts about our past; and involuntary future thoughts. This means dwelling (usually negatively) on the past or fears of that unknown future. Many people compare this to intrusive thoughts of conditions such as schizophrenia or OCD. The main difference is that with ADHD these intrusive thoughts are usually based on real past events or possible future consequences (a bit like rejection sensitive dysphoria), although often with the most negative possible interpretation or expectations of what might happen. This is probably a form of anxiety that can be caused by or coexist with ADHD.

Again, in everyday life, most people experience involuntary thoughts about their past and future events in response to cues in the environment (such as a photo or the smell of food). Yet, most people are NOT often flooded by these thoughts. This is because most people have the ability to inhibit or control these thoughts to stop them from popping up. But not most people with ADHD.

Impulsivity

If you aren't just inattentive-type ADHD (what they used to call ADD), you will notice that alongside hyperactivity in the diagnostic criteria for ADHD sits impulsivity. The concept of impulsivity covers a wide range of actions and reactions.

ADHD UNPACKED

These are the types of things we do in life that may have been poorly thought through, prematurely acted on, or a bit risky. As with inattention, almost everyone has been impulsive at some point in their lives (and it can even be a positive thing in small doses, or we wouldn't ever ask someone on a date). For every human, who among us can honestly say that they have never had one last drink or bite of cake? Who hasn't bought something online on a whim or had a one-night stand? Perhaps Alex for that last one, but the point is that *sometimes* being impulsive leads to bad things happening, but not always. A little bit of impulsivity can be an attractive thing. But a lot of unregulated impulsivity can be quite damaging.

In about 70 per cent of adults with ADHD, impulsive behaviour is a pain in the arse. This is our description of the results of years of psychological research. In ADHD, this impulsivity is typically not a major advantage most of the time. The lack of internal brakes that would normally restrict us from impulse spending, from interrupting people when they are speaking, or from failing to walk away and think about a response before emailing our boss calling them a 'thieving [expletive deleted]' (as James once did), can cause problems at home, at work and in relationships. The fact that James didn't get sacked for that one is still a surprise.

Having internal brakes is the ability to inhibit our responses to thoughts and actions. Both hyperactivity and impulsivity are thought to occur because of a lack of 'response inhibition'. This includes our ability to stop a behaviour (or thought) or to *prepare* to stop a behaviour (or thought) even when prewarned that it might happen. So even if we know that something is going to happen, we can still react impulsively. This means that looking for common triggers and avoiding them where possible is a well-documented coping strategy for adults with ADHD. It just isn't always that easy.

Diagnostically, as with inattention, there are also nine symptoms of hyperactivity/impulsiveness. These are (boringly) listed below – have a look at Chapter 6 if you want a reminder of the full diagnostic criteria for ADHD. As with the inattentive symptoms, most people might say that they recognise these in themselves from time to time, but if five out of the nine symptoms occur very often, and make your life difficult, they can indicate ADHD. If you have ADHD, this is like the worst Christmas list of things you don't want to do all day, every day. It is the 'socks and a cardigan' of psychological symptoms.

DSMV hyperactive-impulsive type ADHD symptoms

1. Often fidgets with or taps hands or feet, or squirms in seat.

2. Often leaves seat in situations when remaining seated is expected.

3. Often runs about or climbs in situations where it is not appropriate (adolescents or adults may be limited to feeling restless).

4. Often unable to play or take part in leisure activities quietly.

5. Is often 'on-the-go' acting as if 'driven by a motor.'

6. Often talks excessively.

7. Often blurts out an answer before a question has been completed.

8. Often has trouble waiting their turn.

9. Often interrupts or intrudes on others (e.g. butts into conversations or games).

You may not be surprised to hear that yet again, as with attention, the prefrontal cortex of the brain is involved in hyperactivity. Along with a brain area called the striatum, the planning of movements and actions occurs here. 'Striatum' just means furrowed or wrinkled and it is a part of that basal ganglia bit that controls movement. Ganglia mean collections of nerves, while basal means 'on the ground', so the stress of learning complicated words such as 'basal ganglia striatum' seems particularly pointless given that it means 'wrinkly bit of brain on the bottom'.

SIT STILL AND DON'T INTERRUPT!

SUMMARY

Although there are three types of ADHD, between half and two thirds of us have hyperactivity and impulsivity in our type. Many people dismiss the hyperactivity part of their ADHD because they have either internalised it or they haven't quite understood what the rest of the world is like. This is especially common when we start comparing ourselves to our families, many of whom share our ADHD traits; it looks like it is very common to never comfortably sit still. Who among us have had family members who confidently and incorrectly tell us, 'Everyone is like that'?

The reason it is important to think about how you can work with your traits is that they can make many elements of life very uncomfortable (such as learning quietly at college or university, relaxing with a partner, cinema trips or work meetings). By recognising and communicating these difficulties, we can start to compromise. Or at the very least, we can learn to understand that it isn't that we don't like the people around us or the subject of the meeting, but rather that we might need to have breaks, walk around a bit or find a pen that doesn't make a really loud clicking sound at the cinema when we press it a hundred times during *Oppenheimer*. Or *Barbie*.

Whether we identify as a more hyperactive/impulsive type or present with significant inattention, a huge element of ADHD is how our brains struggle with acting or thinking in the way that we would intellectually choose. To align those things, we need our long-term intentions to match our subconscious brain's need to clearly feel a short-term emotional reward for doing it. The next chapter will take a closer look at this idea of reward and why both reward and dopamine are always so heavily linked to ADHD.

CHAPTER 10

Reward and ADHD

For any of us to do something, we have to persuade our brain that it is worth doing. That we will get a 'reward' for doing it. This doesn't have to be a literal reward, such as money or a treat. It can be a positive feeling (or the removal of a negative feeling such as guilt). In order to do any task at all, our brain needs to feel that reward will come. It does this by using a connected group of brain areas called (imaginatively) the 'reward centre'.

Evidence suggests that people with ADHD don't have a properly working reward system in their brain.[54] This means we are probably less able to feel the potential reward for starting or doing a task, even if intellectually, we really want to do it. A common misconception is that we don't want to do these things when, in fact, we are facing a sort of paralysis that we often can't explain ourselves. This can be true even if we know that a specific task is objectively important for us, our job or even our partner. This not only makes some tasks very difficult to do, but trying to communicate that mental block can be equally difficult.

It is exhausting. We often have to push ourselves to achieve what most people would consider to be a simple, small job if our brain doesn't feel the clear short-term reward of doing it. For us to mentally overcome that lack of anticipated reward takes a lot of energy. When people say that it just takes 'willpower' to do these things, it feels like we have run a mile, only to be told, 'All you need is willpower to run another hundred miles.' It doesn't work like that. With ADHD, the physical and mental cost of pushing through that lack of reward is very high.

What is reward?

So, what exactly do we mean when we refer to this feeling of reward? If you want a big picture sentence, we would say: '*Reward is a feeling that attracts us and motivates us to approach something and consume it in some way.*' (Not just eat it.) Essentially, it is the drive to do something, and this doesn't have to be because it makes us happy. Reward isn't the same as happiness.

We have evolved this need to feel rewarded to learn things about life. It helps us remember which trees have the best fruit on, for example, or which people make us feel safe – these rewards are important to recall. We also need to remember things that won't leave us rewarded and learn to avoid them (such as velvet, which is a material that should be banned).

It is easy to describe feeling rewarded, right? You just ... erm ... you feel happy? Is that it? Happy? Or is it content and peaceful? Or is it just that some mental itch has been

REWARD AND ADHD

scratched? OK, maybe it is the anticipation of getting something – or is it when you have already got that thing? What if someone else gives you a reward? Is that the same?

It isn't easy to describe reward, and that confusion comes from the fact that it isn't just one thing, even to your own brain. A useful way to describe those differences is to split reward into three main types: reward receipt, anticipated reward and uncertain anticipated reward.

Reward receipt

The simplest type of reward is the feeling of pleasure or satisfaction when we get or do something. This is called the reward receipt and probably isn't much different for the general population compared to those of us with ADHD.[55] Having said that, the research is mixed on this one, and there are one or two studies suggesting that the brains of people with ADHD don't get enough pleasure sensations from things (less reward receipt). The problem with those studies is that people with ADHD are also more likely to have a condition called anhedonia (which means not feeling as much joy). If we imagine going on a shopping trip, this simple type of reward receipt is that feeling of having the item you have shopped for – let's say a cardigan. They even give you a receipt, which makes that type of reward easy to remember.

Anticipated reward

The second type of reward is the anticipation of reward, and this is often a more powerful driver of motivation for people to do something than reward receipt. Being honest, what is a bigger motivator when you go on a shopping trip? Is it getting home with something you have bought, or is it the anticipation of getting a bargain when you go shopping? Very often, it is that second one. This type of reward, the anticipation of reward, does seem to be an even stronger factor for motivation in adults with ADHD than ordinary people, overriding other, often more sensible, long-term plans or choices. There is quite a lot of evidence that the part of the brain that anticipates reward is less active (including lots of dopamine-based systems) in people with ADHD.[56,57]

Uncertain anticipated reward

The last and arguably most dangerous type of reward takes us back to that shopping trip one more time. Imagine that bargain you want. Now imagine you are not sure if it will be available in the first place. It might be sold out. You don't know for sure if you are going to get it. This uncertainty can be a yet more powerful driver to go shopping in the first place than the other two reward types, particularly for people with ADHD.

This is called uncertain anticipatory reward and appears to cause the highest levels of dopamine activity in people in general. One experiment that showed this scanned the brains of people while they were gambling (whether they had a gambling problem or not). What was very surprising is that it didn't seem to be the winning that activated the most dopamine, or even the anticipation of winning. It was the uncertainty of winning at all.[58] The uncertainty of getting a reward. These big companies know this. They make gambling easy on your phone, offer free little games where you might get a prize or harmless apps with pull-down buttons to see if you have a new notification. They abuse it horrifically, causing damage that disproportionately affects those of us with ADHD, for which they should be ashamed.

Getting a reward is a feeling that people with ADHD crave. Anticipating that reward is even more of a motivating factor and that uncertain anticipation of reward is stronger still. But why is that?

The strong link between reward and ADHD

Loads of brain networks link reward with actions, and these pretty much all seem to be affected in adults with ADHD. However, the key part is the 'reward centre' of the brain or 'mesocorticolimbic system' (which really just means 'middle-outside-edge' bit but in a sort of hybrid Greek-Latin mixture). This reward centre is a network that includes several areas of the brain (unsurprisingly, you will find those areas in the middle, outside and edge bits) related to feeling emotions and executive functions. Executive functions are the planning and organising parts of the brain that enable us to chase those rewards, and ADHD people can struggle with these a lot. We will talk a lot more about executive functions in Chapter 12.

Dopamine is central to the perception and processing of reward[59] and that whole reward centre network of the brain functions differently in ADHD in a few ways. This includes having lower dopamine activity levels, differences in dopamine receptor function and a delayed response to potential rewards. This means that we often tend to act on immediate, small rewards over larger but delayed rewards (this is an executive function called 'delay discounting').

Short-term rewards, delay discounting and delayed gratification

This last thing we need to remember about reward and ADHD is that our brain tends to need to see the emotional reward in a really short or even immediate time frame. There is a tendency for modern society to get the blame for all sorts of things that are basic human nature. One of them is that we are the 'instant-gratification society'. We are told that modern society wants everything right now or not at all. That we can't save up for things or wait for good things to come. There may be some truth in this, but as a criticism it is really quite harsh. All humans have delay discounting: feeling less motivation for rewards the further these are away from us. This feeling also seems to be exceptionally strong in people with ADHD. It might be that we need to feel stronger emotions to trigger the motivation to act (so the reward has to be closer to us in time) or it might be that we just don't perceive time well so we don't feel it if the reward is farther away.

In terms of just waiting for things (or saving up for things), people with ADHD are probably going to experience a stronger urge to 'have it now'. Delayed gratification isn't our strong point. From a practical perspective, we have to find a short-term reason to persuade our brains to delay gratification. But that isn't the only type of reward. What if the delayed gratification was bigger than having the reward now? What if you got a bigger reward for waiting?

REWARD AND ADHD

Let's say we offered you a small reward now, such as a cake (a nice one). What if we could offer you a bigger cake a year from now? Which would you choose? Probably the cake now, right? This is where the strength of delayed gratification gets complicated (although the oppositional defiance common to ADHD means we know that both of us would probably say, 'I don't like cake', or something. Try to restrict that urge if possible).

To look at your own response to delay, try changing cake to something you would like more than cake. What if we offered you that bigger reward tomorrow instead of right now? Or five minutes from now? The further away the reward, the harder it is to wait. What if we make it a bigger difference between the reward now and the reward for waiting? A cake now – or a thousand pounds in one year? Easier right? But with ADHD, this ability to wait for a reward and the power of an increase in the value of that reward is also less effective. Not impossible – just less effective.[60]

Dopamine and reward

In terms of HOW the neurotransmitters such as dopamine work in our brain's reward centre, it is horribly complicated and still far from clear to science (and even less clear to us). There are some oversimplified models that you might have seen describing dopamine as the 'reward chemical', and maybe also describing serotonin as the 'happiness hormone' or noradrenaline as the 'only driver of fear or anger'? This isn't correct.

Dopamine is central to reward in the brain, but it is much more complicated than saying dopamine equals reward. One way to visualise this is to think of brain chemicals such as dopamine and serotonin (and others) acting like the keys on a piano playing different notes. You can press those keys together at the same time, alone and at different times, or with different strengths, and you can create whole chords and even virtuoso musical arrangements with just a few notes. You could do that arrangement in the key of C, for example, but that wouldn't mean that the entire musical piece was just played with one C note, even if C is central to the music. It is the same with dopamine and reward; dopamine is central but not sufficient to explain our reward behaviour. There are lots of other factors.

Motivation

Motivation is the process that initiates, guides and maintains our goal-oriented behaviours. Biologically speaking, motivation is a series of neurological processes that initiate behaviour and then both directs and sustains that behaviour towards a specific goal. Motivation describes how we start, continue with and finish any task (or how we stop doing those things). We have included it in this chapter because motivation requires the brain's reward system. Think about the reward you need to motivate yourself to start something, and to not get distracted while doing that thing and to get that thing finished – you can see why motivation and feeling rewarded are so linked.

When an activity results in a reward or the anticipation of a reward (uncertain or otherwise), dopamine activity increases (not just dopamine), which reinforces that behaviour and motivates us to repeat it. Put simply, motivation often comes from reward.

Types of motivation can differ for people with ADHD

Motivation can be separated into 'intrinsic' motivation (from within) and 'extrinsic' motivation (from outside). An example of intrinsic motivation might be the drive to study for an exam because you want to get a good grade (or not feel bad about getting a poor grade). Examples of extrinsic motivation might be engaging with a task because the deadline is tomorrow or doing things for other people because you like those people or are afraid of them telling you off (or both).

If the reward centre works differently in ADHD, it would follow that motivation for people with ADHD might be different as well. And it is, or at least it usually is for many of us, and research can back this up (for a change). Firstly, people living with ADHD appear to be more likely to have 'amotivation'.[61] Amotivation is the lack or absence of the drive to engage in any activity. So, if you have ADHD, you may be less motivated to work towards goals you have identified (even if you know these are important priorities). Again, this isn't about willpower or 'wanting it'; it is a lack of internal drive to engage with a task, even if you want to. The same study also suggests that people with ADHD tend to have higher levels of 'extrinsic' motivation than 'intrinsic' motivation (not all of us, remember — science is rarely so black and white). This means that many of us are more motivated to do things if there is external accountability, or a hard deadline, than we are to do things for ourselves with nobody watching.

This is one of the reasons why many adults with ADHD use the 'buddy system' of doing a task in the same room as somebody else (a buddy) even if they are not actually helping. It seems to provide a feeling of external accountability without the demotivating factor of somebody checking on you.

You might notice that the motivation for some people to study for an exam might be intrinsic (wanting to do well), whereas others might study for extrinsic reasons (making a teacher happy, for example). This is one reason why moving from the structure of school to college, employment or university can cause serious difficulties for adults with ADHD who are struggling to find the same motivation.

According to a study published in 2022, motivation levels in people living with ADHD were improved when their needs of autonomy (feeling you have a choice), relatedness (feeling connected to others and a sense of belonging), and competence (mastery or successfulness in your activity) were met.[62] For people living with ADHD, meeting these needs may require different approaches than those needed to motivate a person who doesn't have ADHD, especially in workplaces and educational institutes that have a rigid set of expectations. Rules put in place 'because we've always done it like this' can be very unhelpful for adults with ADHD.

SUMMARY

There is a difference between feeling happy about getting rewarded and being motivated to do something because you will feel rewarded afterwards. ADHD seems to be strongly linked to seeking out tasks that offer a higher reward in the relatively short-term. Being angry with ourselves for not being able to start or finish tasks is unhelpful if our brain can't see the short-term emotional reward for doing them. This isn't a simple case of willpower, and it isn't enough to say 'because it needs to be done'.

The only way to try and deal with this is to build tasks that are typically within your own experience of things you usually find rewarding. You might have to write down the times when you have felt that, because we often find it difficult to know what we think and feel, especially when asked under pressure. Another way to start is to try and interpret the tasks you want to achieve in a way that will make you feel good. For example, try writing S.M.A.R.T objectives for tasks with a positive outcome on how you feel or how the people around you feel. (See Chapter 16 for how to set S.M.A.R.T goals.)

ADHD can feel like a lifetime of struggling to do things that everyone else feels are really simple to do. For us to get important things done, we need to prioritise intellectually but align those priorities with the emotional side of our brain as well. We need to feel that the task is worth doing in the short term, and we need to be aware of the challenges ADHD provides in regulating our emotions in the first place. The next chapter looks at that link between ADHD and emotions in a lot more detail.

CHAPTER 11

Emotions and rejection in ADHD

Almost everyone we know in our community seems to struggle more with the dysregulation of emotions than with any other aspect of their ADHD. Despite this, the name 'attention deficit hyperactivity disorder' makes no reference to the emotional side of ADHD. Managing the core symptoms of inattention and hyperactivity and impulsive behaviour (for those of us who are a triple threat) is difficult enough without having to also try to manage our often-unpredictable emotions.

This side of ADHD manifests itself in two main ways: emotional dysregulation and rejection sensitive dysphoria (or ED and RSD for short). In some people, there are other issues, including alexithymia (sadly not named after Alex) and anhedonia but they are probably extra embuggerances we have to deal with on top of ADHD.

In this chapter, we will have a look at all of these key emotional components of ADHD, explaining why they happen, the impact they can have on our day-to-day lives and what we can start to do about them.

Emotional Dysregulation (ED)

This isn't just about strong emotions. How most people respond to something emotionally isn't something they are always consciously aware of. But if that emotional response doesn't seem to be consistent with the majority of people, you could say that you were having emotional dysregulation. To understand this, it is helpful to first understand emotional regulation in general, which is one of the 'executive functions' that we will be discussing more in the next chapter.

Emotions are often confused with hormones, feelings and moods, but these are different. Emotions are generally how people deal with issues, people or situations they find personally significant.[63] The emotions we experience are thought to have three components: our subjective experience (the thing that we respond to), a physiological response (how our body reacts) and a behavioural response (how we behave).

We all have emotional reactions many times every day. Unlike most other animals, we have a higher ability to manage and respond more appropriately to an emotional experience in a 'socially acceptable' and flexible manner. This emotional regulation is a major part of human society, but the words 'socially acceptable' do a lot of the heavy lifting in that last sentence. The way in which people are

EMOTIONS AND REJECTION IN ADHD

expected to respond to life's events is, to a large degree, a social construct. We are expected to respond emotionally to some events (such as a wedding or funeral) in a certain way and usually very differently to the way in which we respond to other apparently less important events. Responding emotionally in a way that is expected in your society is called having a predictable emotional response. In ADHD, our emotional responses are often far less predictable and often not seen as 'socially acceptable'.

We both experience this often. One of the examples of emotional dysregulation we talk about quite a lot on our podcast happened not that long ago. James had an early train home from somewhere, so he stopped to get a fast-food breakfast from a well-known clown-based establishment (other clown-based burgers are available. Probably). It was one of the newer self-service restaurants, and the printed-out ticket from the touch screen read 'Order number 89'. While waiting patiently (like a Tasmanian devil might), James saw someone with a later order (number 91) being served their food. Instead of thinking there was a reason for this, James lost his shit at the poor member of staff serving. As he furiously argued, flecks of spittle painting the counter, he thought to himself, 'WHAT ARE YOU DOING?' Once he finally got his meal, he sat down only to find that he had been given the wrong order. Instead of acting in a 'normal' way, James went back and doubled down, venting as if someone had kicked his dog. James can never go back into that fast-food restaurant again. Or several other shops (for unrelated reasons). This was a clear overreaction, but it wasn't planned or desired – it just happened.

This lack of control or predictability over emotional responses can be problematic because emotional regulation is important for many reasons. Chief among those are the maintenance of both personal and professional relationships, coping with stresses throughout our lives and also the general effect of those emotions on stabilising our mental health.

If someone responds to a fairly run-of-the-mill life event with an explosive emotional reaction, such as James and his bacon and egg muffin, this can cause friction in their life, especially for their own self-esteem and within personal and professional relationships. Equally, if a big life event happens and the emotional response to it is just 'meh', this apparent apathy could also cause friction within those relationships and within ourselves. Alex has never cried over the death of a loved one in his life, not because he didn't love them, but because he didn't have that emotional reaction when it happened. There is no 'reason' why not. It is just a different emotional response to one that is expected (he did cry when he was given the wrong potatoes at dinner once though, so the humiliation of that is perfectly easy to live with). This doesn't really affect anyone else but (until learning how to accept ADHD) it had quite a profound negative effect on how Alex sees himself as a part of a loving family.

Expressing emotions differently to the expectations of society is a problem for many of us, but it is far more problematic when the emotional response we have doesn't match our own personal expectations and values. That can be an incredible source of shame. Whether it is road rage

EMOTIONS AND REJECTION IN ADHD

or an argument with a partner that feels very important at the time but not so important later, this can be inconsistent with how we see ourselves and who we want to be. We are often asked if we 'are ADHD' or 'have ADHD', and this is an example of the latter. For us, this is ADHD stopping us being who we really are.

Emotional regulation isn't really a question of trying to suppress or control our emotions all of the time (we can't easily do that, and it probably isn't very healthy to suppress the feelings themselves).[64] It is more about managing our emotions effectively. It is far more important to start to acknowledge, understand and interpret our emotional responses (and their triggers) in more constructive ways.

Your emotions are literally all in your mind

As with other executive functions, emotional regulation is broadly controlled by the parts of the brain that often develop slightly differently in people with ADHD and therefore function slightly differently as well. We introduced quite a few ridiculous names for bits of the brain in Chapter 3, and several of those are involved in emotional regulation. Some of the main ones are the prefrontal cortex (very front of the fronty bit), the amygdala (from the Greek word for almond, because of the shape of this brain part, not its flavour, probably) and the hippocampus (also from the Greek, this time for 'seahorse', and again because of the shape of this part of the brain, not the flavour).

Brain scan studies show that emotional dysregulation (including in adults with ADHD) is largely due to these

ADHD UNPACKED

brain areas not being built or working quite like they do in most people. This biological brain difference heavily influences the behavioural difference in modulating emotional responses (both too much and too little of an emotional reaction).

For people who are combined type ADHD, or the small group who may be purely hyperactive/impulsive type ADHD, impulsivity also extends to emotional responses. Adults with ADHD might react more quickly and intensely to life's events, having a weaker ability to step back, pause and think before responding. This can then lead to the exaggerated or understated emotional reactions that can be seen as inappropriate or overwhelming.

As if this weren't complicated enough, about 80 per cent of adults with ADHD have a coexisting condition (and around 50 per cent have more than one). We personally call this ADHD+ (or ADHD plus, covered a lot more in Chapter 15) and this can severely compound the difficulties faced in emotional regulation. For example, having anxiety can heighten emotional responses to any event or thought. Depression and alcohol use disorder can both affect the ability to experience and express positive emotions.[65]

The challenges of ADHD and emotional dysregulation can cause serious social and professional difficulties. Problems managing, interpreting and expressing emotions can result in conflicts, misunderstandings and social isolation. It is difficult enough to navigate personal, familial or professional relationships when you have the core symptoms of ADHD, but when you add in unpredictable and 'socially

EMOTIONS AND REJECTION IN ADHD

inappropriate' emotional responses, this adds even more difficulty in establishing and maintaining relationships at any level. Saying or doing things that may be regretted later on is often not received well by others. We will talk a lot more about ADHD and relationships in Chapter 13.

Emotional dysregulation doesn't just impact those around us; it can have a huge impact on how we view ourselves. Emotional outbursts or the inability to react 'appropriately' in emotional situations can lead to feelings of guilt, shame and low self-esteem. The feeling of 'Why did I say that?' often leads to self-loathing, which can further impact mental health. If you love or have a strong relationship with someone, and your actions upset them, it is understandable that you may dislike yourself for upsetting that person.

In our experience, we often have strong emotional reactions that seem very real at the time but then lose significance minutes or hours later. This can be frustrating when you have argued a point quite strongly that you no longer care about. It can sometimes make it harder to advocate for things you do care about in the future. This feeling of shame and regret can be particularly difficult to deal with for people who are undiagnosed with ADHD, as they are less likely to understand the reason for their response.

What can we do about emotional dysregulation?

Although we can't choose our emotional reactions, with diagnosis and support we can start moving towards emotional acceptance of ADHD. When you accept that these feelings are part of your neurological make-up, it can help to diminish this shame somewhat. So, although acceptance can't control those emotions, it can help us to interpret them more kindly, which can reduce the chances of having unwanted emotional reactions in the future. Remember: ADHD is a reason, not an excuse. What this means is that we all of course know that ADHD doesn't provide complete freedom to act without self-control at all times, but it does explain why we sometimes act in a way we don't wish to.

Emotional dysregulation in the workplace

In the workplace, emotional dysregulation can manifest as overreactions to feedback, difficulty handling stress and perceived unfairness, and challenges in teamwork. Some people with ADHD report their own emotional dysregulation as an advantage in certain jobs, such as paramedics with an inappropriately low emotional response to accidents. Unfortunately, we can't always predict when we will have differing levels of emotional response.

For most of us, emotional dysregulation can hamper career progress and job satisfaction. If you think about most workplace environments, whether enduring annual appraisals or receiving feedback on work that is produced, it is easy to see that there are plenty of opportunities for emotional dysregulation. It is also easy to see in this context that if people don't understand ADHD, or don't know that a colleague has ADHD, they could be frustrated or upset by an emotional response that they either didn't predict or that they don't think is appropriate.

EMOTIONS AND REJECTION IN ADHD

This is where it is important to say that it is absolutely valid for people without ADHD to be upset at an emotional response that affects them, if they don't feel it is appropriate. This is natural. However, it is also completely valid for somebody with ADHD to not have complete control over their emotional responses. This can easily create a situation in which there is friction with no blame to attach, leaving both people feeling frustrated and rather negative.

One way to approach this (as well as clear communication) is to explore strategies and tools that can help people manage their emotions more healthily. This could include therapy such as CBT (or relationship counselling) or talking to professionals (such as an ADHD-informed coach). These tools can help to develop skills for identifying, understanding and managing our emotions and their common triggers. Some people find the ADHD medication can also help in the management of their emotional dysregulation. While this doesn't happen for everyone, medication can improve impulse control, which in turn can aid better emotional regulation. As always, ADHD medication is a personal choice.

If you can find a way to engage with them (and James and I laugh about how boring this can be), mindfulness meditation and relaxation techniques may help you develop a greater awareness of your emotional state and help to prepare for situations that may be a trigger for an emotional response. This can help to promote a calm and measured response to emotional stimuli. Alex tends to make meditation and mindfulness 'ADHD-friendly', which means combining breathing and reflection with other activities (anything you like to do that isn't operating heavy machinery) and significantly shortening the duration of meditation (sometimes to as little as thirty seconds to a minute).

Reducing stressors (such as alcohol and drugs) and accessing physical exercise can also help with these emotional dysregulation responses, but then we all already know that. If we had to choose a single approach, the best support for emotional dysregulation is other people. Having a strong support system of family, friends and colleagues who understand ADHD and are better able to identify when we might not be in control of our emotional responses is incredibly helpful. It is also, sadly, not that common. The lack of societal awareness and acceptance of ADHD means most people don't really know what it is, and almost certainly don't know it extends to our emotions. These support systems can be anything from agreeing in advance a non-verbal signal for when we are feeling overwhelmed (Alex raises a hand) or a pre-agreed conversation about when we need to leave a room without explanation for a few minutes that won't then be interpreted as 'storming off angrily'.

Rejection sensitive dysphoria (RSD)

This is a big one. So many people with ADHD hear about rejection sensitivity disorder and realise they have had this their entire lives. It can be quite destabilising. RSD isn't always easy to explain because almost no one likes being rejected; but with ADHD, the response to rejection feels like it has been dialled up much more than might normally be expected.

EMOTIONS AND REJECTION IN ADHD

RSD isn't a recognised medical mental health disorder (unlike ADHD), but can be described as a psychological condition in which an individual has a hugely heightened emotional response to being rejected, criticised or ignored. RSD also includes someone *thinking* that they have been rejected, criticised or ignored. To make things worse, RSD also commonly kicks in when *we think we are going to be* rejected, criticised or ignored, even if it doesn't seem likely at all. Even if, intellectually, we know that we probably won't face that rejection.

Most people probably feel hurt when they are rejected, but if you have ADHD and RSD, even the potential for future rejection *hurts so much more*. Alex often describes this as being like 'emotional sunburn' (but he probably stole that from someone). If the pain of rejection is like a sharp slap on the back that naturally hurts a little bit, then rejection with RSD feels like being slapped on the back when you have serious sunburn. It can be incredibly painful, and we will do almost anything to avoid that pain.

This means RSD can have a profound impact on emotional well-being and interpersonal relationships. Rejection sensitivity isn't just feeling a bit upset after a social snub or criticism; it involves an intense, often overwhelming emotional (and physical) reaction that can include feelings of anxiety, sadness and even anger. It can lead to a heightened vigilance to the smallest potential rejection cues and a tendency to perceive rejection in ambiguous situations. This can often lead us down one of two paths: pathologically avoiding any situation in which we may be rejected (social withdrawal), or people please, where we spend huge amounts of emotional and physical labour to avoid rejection, often becoming someone who says yes to every request – because if you say yes, it is more difficult to be rejected. These reactions can be disproportionate to the actual situation and can have lasting impacts on an individual's mental health and social functioning.

Why do people with ADHD have RSD?

Surprisingly, even though pretty much every adult with ADHD reports an increased sensitivity to rejection, there is very little research on the subject, probably because adult ADHD is relatively new. There are converging biological and social issues that probably contribute. Firstly, part of RSD is a form of emotional dysregulation (which is why we are talking about it in this chapter), and the parts of the brain that process emotions, especially negative ones, both look and act differently in people with ADHD.

Where it gets more complex is that on top of our biological brain difference, people with ADHD are more likely to have faced trauma and rejection from an early age.[66] It has been estimated that around 50–60 per cent of ADHD children experience rejection by their peers, and even children who were diagnosed with ADHD at the age of four had more rejection from other children by the age of six.[67] Although the theory of rejection sensitivity, which was developed in 1996,[68] suggested that the early life rejection is the main cause and that RSD develops as a result of early, prolonged or acute experiences of rejection, that was decades before research into adult ADHD was meaningful, so it probably isn't the whole story. It is true that adults with ADHD tend to have experienced many

EMOTIONS AND REJECTION IN ADHD

actual rejections and criticisms throughout their lives, often related to their ADHD symptoms. These experiences can lead to the development of a heightened sensitivity to rejection, as people come to anticipate and overreact to potential rejections in the future.

At the same time, RSD could be seen as a form of emotional dysregulation, which is part of the biology of ADHD itself. It isn't at all clear whether adults of ADHD have rejection sensitivity because of the different way in which their brains develop, or if rejection sensitivity develops because of a lifetime of feeling different, being rejected and receiving criticism.

Whatever causes it, the impact of RSD in adults with ADHD can't easily be understated. As with emotional dysregulation, perceiving and anticipating rejection can lead to difficulties in forming and maintaining relationships (both personal and professional). Withdrawing from social interactions to avoid potential rejection can lead to isolation. RSD in the workplace can manifest as an exaggerated response to feedback or criticism, leading to conflicts with colleagues, anxiety about job performance (even if that performance isn't a problem) and the impulsive urge to leave a job without good reason because of the strength of the feeling of rejection or criticism. James once immediately left a job as a bartender because he wasn't praised for bringing the tables in from the storage area the night before, but another bartender was. When asked why he was leaving, James was so embarrassed that he said he had a virus. When asked which one, he replied, 'They don't know.'

This story is an example of how living with RSD means constantly anticipating and overreacting to rejection, which can then lead to choices that are not in our own interests and can also erode self-esteem and self-worth. This is probably one of many reasons why adults with ADHD often develop a negative self-image, believing they are inherently flawed or unlikeable. The urge for Alex and James to make jokes about each other being both flawed and unlikeable at this point was very strong but we have resisted.

RSD can even have an impact on our sleep. Many of us will lie awake at night, preparing for a conversation with somebody where we feel rejection or criticism may occur, going through every possible permutation of how that conversation could go, only for it to go absolutely smoothly the following day (or not even happen at all). The fear of that conversation going badly is enough to lead to a ridiculous level of over-preparation. Also, that conversation inside our heads isn't a dialogue; it is a monologue. We are often making biased assumptions that the other person involved in that conversation will definitely reject us, and therefore mentally this is what we prepare for. A friend of Alex's (we'll call her Maria) once reminded him that in those imaginary conversations he was, in fact, talking to himself. This was accurate but hurtful.

As ADHD coaches, we often work with adults for whom RSD is the most prominent issue causing their challenges. This is one of the most difficult aspects of ADHD to manage. As with emotional dysregulation, psychotherapy or coaching can be a practical tool for some people to help identify situations that may trigger RSD. It can also help us to start putting strategies in place to be able to better deal with the situation in the

EMOTIONS AND REJECTION IN ADHD

moment, and to genuinely question a situation afterwards. This can help us to work out whether rejection or criticism actually occurred, or if we just misunderstood the situation.

All of this feels like an advert for ADHD coaching from ADHD coaches. It really isn't. We recommend you find much better ones than us. You can also coach yourself, if you can find the time to sit and think about your goals and strengths. That could be better than us, quite frankly.

Alexithymia

The third emotional gift that ADHD gives many of us is alexithymia. This term was coined in the 1970s and refers to a condition in which somebody has difficulty in identifying, describing and working with their own emotions. This is not a widely known condition, and not everyone with ADHD has it. It is thought that around 10 per cent of the general population may have alexithymia, but in the ADHD population this number increases to as high as 40 per cent.

Alexithymia has got nothing to do with the name Alex (disappointingly). 'Lexythymia' (without an 'A' at the front) means describing your mind in Latin (the word is in Latin; it doesn't mean you have to explain your feelings in Latin). So 'A-lexythymia' means not being able to do that. If you ask yourself to describe your state of mind (in your own language), how well can you do that?

If you struggle with identifying, verbalising or analysing your feelings (either emotional or physical feelings, such as describing pain), you may be experiencing alexithymia. This could also include difficulties in understanding the experiences and feelings inside your own mind and in your ability to express those feelings to others. What does this look like in real life? It could be having difficulty identifying feelings such as hunger or sadness, but it could also be a problem differentiating between the range of common emotions. There is a running joke in our community that the most common and accurate ADHD answer to 'How are you?' is 'I really don't know.' Other types of alexithymia might include:

- difficulties distinguishing between our emotional feelings and the bodily sensations of emotional arousal (which isn't as rude as it sounds, meaning having strong emotions like anger)

- difficulty finding words to describe feelings to other people (James has to interpret his wife's descriptions of illness such as 'fizzy stomach')

- constricted imagination (both in images and content)

- a thought content characterised by a preoccupation with the minute details of external events (especially when trying to write a book of this size and focusing on a bee in the garden, for example)

On top of all that, people with a high alexithymia level can also have difficulties in recognising and empathising with the emotional states of other people. Studies looking at the ability to identify facial expressions of emotion in adults with ADHD have shown that ADHDers perform worse on

EMOTIONS AND REJECTION IN ADHD

facial emotion recognition (for example, showing someone a photo of a happy face and asking them which emotion this is) and can make more mistakes when matching facial emotions with the appropriate context. None of these are obligatory, by the way. We are always just suggesting different ways in which people with ADHD might be affected. This last one also might reflect the increased incidence of autistic spectrum condition and autistic traits that coexist with ADHD.

Both ADHD and alexithymia involve irregularities in brain regions responsible for emotional processing and regulation, and again involve our favourite brain parts, the prefrontal cortex and the almond-flavoured amygdala. These differences in brain regions can impact how people with ADHD perceive and process emotional information, contributing to alexithymic traits. As well as the biological causes of alexithymia, adults with ADHD may also have experienced difficulties in social interactions from a young age. These early challenges can affect social learning, particularly in understanding and interpreting emotions, both in themselves and in others. This lack of social-emotional learning can also contribute to the development of alexithymic traits. So, it could be part biology, part social. Nature and nurture combined. We don't know.

What we do know is that having alexithymia is more than just a quirk and can have far-reaching implications. If you are struggling to understand or express emotions, alexithymia can lead to misunderstandings and conflicts in personal relationships. People with ADHD and alexithymia may appear indifferent or emotionally distant (even if they are burning inside), impacting their ability to form close and supportive relationships. In the workplace, alexithymia can look like a lack of emotional intelligence; it can impact on our expectations of teamwork, leadership and job satisfaction. We might struggle with tasks that require emotional understanding and empathy, such as customer service or team management.

Being unable to understand and work with emotions can also hinder personal growth and self-awareness. Adults with ADHD and alexithymia may struggle with self-reflection and self-improvement efforts, which often rely on emotional insight. On the plus side, neither of us have this (meta-joke).

Anhedonia

Have you ever sat and watched a sunset, feeling serene? Or held a newborn child and felt pure joy? James hasn't. While he has seen many sunsets, and held at least five children, James has anhedonia. Anhedonia refers to a reduced ability, or inability, to experience pleasure from activities that are usually found enjoyable, such as social events, food or sex (not all together). Anhedonia is often associated with mental health conditions, including major depressive disorder and substance use disorders, but it is also sometimes found in people with ADHD.

Of these four emotional issues, anhedonia has the least research or statistics behind it. Many people with ADHD have coexisting mood disorders or substance use

EMOTIONS AND REJECTION IN ADHD

disorders, so it is difficult to establish at the moment whether any link between ADHD and anhedonia comes from ADHD itself or if it is more likely because of the increased chances of having coexisting conditions. Depression or anxiety often include symptoms of anhedonia, for example. Therefore, anhedonia in someone with ADHD might be a feature of a co-occurring depressive disorder rather than a direct symptom of ADHD itself. It could even be a difficulty recognising pleasure in some people, rather than a lack of enjoyment itself (see alexithymia above).

Having said that, ADHD and those conditions usually associated with anhedonia (such as depression) are all linked to problems in the brain's reward pathways. Most research into anhedonia has shown reduced dopamine activity in the brain as a central feature, and this is shared with ADHD. Dopamine doesn't just regulate feelings of reward; it also contributes towards feelings of pleasure. So, if dopamine doesn't work as well as it should do, this could explain reduced or absent feelings of pleasure in adults with ADHD.

As with the other emotional difficulties in this chapter, anhedonia can significantly affect a person's quality of life, leading to difficulties in maintaining relationships, pursuing goals or finding motivation in daily tasks.

SUMMARY

ADHD is much more than attention and hyperactivity or impulsivity, and almost all adults with ADHD will have some form of issue with emotions. Emotional dysregulation, rejection sensitivity, alexithymia and anhedonia can be significant challenges for many adults with ADHD. These can all negatively affect social and workplace relationships, self-esteem and positive mental health.

There are many emotional responses that society deems inappropriate, and while social shame can be a big driver, we are not going to allow societal expectations of 'normal' to define us. When our emotional dysregulation hurts the people around us and is outside our own expectations and values, this is a bigger problem, and we want to work on how we can limit this effect.

In addition to diagnosis, treatment and support, accepting the emotional reality of ADHD is a fundamental goal. We might not always be able to control the emotions we are having, or even our emotional response, but we can decide how we interpret that response afterwards. We can communicate and explain to people why that happened and prepare a plan for the next time we feel a similar trigger.

Regulating our emotions is a part of what makes us human. It is also quite complex, as most creatures simply react to their environment – they don't consciously self-regulate very much, and they certainly don't analyse how they are feeling or why! This is one

EMOTIONS AND REJECTION IN ADHD

of the higher order abilities of the human brain, such as organising and planning that is often disrupted in adults with ADHD. These abilities are often grouped together and described as 'executive functions'. In the next chapter, we'll take a look at some of these executive functions and how they can be different in people with ADHD.

CHAPTER 12

Executive Functions and ADHD

At its core, ADHD is an 'executive function disorder'. Executive functions are a set of higher order thinking processes that humans have evolved for everyday goal-directed behaviour. If you want to achieve something, executive functions enable you to plan, coordinate, adjust and engage with whichever tasks are involved. These executive functions also control other cognitive abilities, behaviours and even emotional reactions – similar to how an air traffic controller manages and oversees all the planes' take-offs, landings and movements on the tarmac to ensure safety and efficiency.

Most animals don't tend to think and plan well; they mostly just react to their environment (especially Alex's dog). In humans, the executive functions enable us to consciously start (and crucially stop) doing and saying things even if it isn't our initial reaction. They also enable us to choose how we react to our emotions, to focus on a task or to change tasks even when we are enjoying ourselves. So, when we say that ADHD is an executive function disorder, we mean that the diagnostic symptoms of inattentiveness and hyperactivity/impulsivity seen in ADHD are regulated by those 'higher up' executive functions, and we can really struggle with them.

The parts of the brain that are involved in executive function, and therefore oversee and regulate most of our behaviours, have developed and work differently in adults with ADHD. This means that those executive function brain parts are less able to consistently regulate our behaviour. Experts can't agree on exactly which thinking skills are included in this group of executive functions, but one recent description separates them into *hot* (i.e. reward or mood-related) and *cold* (i.e. purely cognitive) executive functions.[69]

Using this way of describing them, hot executive functions include emotional regulation, reward processing and decision-making (both risky and emotional). Cold executive functions include working memory, inhibitory control, attention control and cognitive flexibility. Some of these issues have already been covered, so in this chapter we will talk specifically about working memory, inhibitory control, cognitive flexibility, emotional decision-making, time management and risk perception. These functions are, again, primarily associated with the prefrontal cortex of the brain, an area we have mentioned many times already. Before we forget, let's start with working memory.

Working memory

Has someone ever read out their telephone number to you, and when you find a pen and paper you can't remember

EXECUTIVE FUNCTIONS AND ADHD

a single digit they mentioned? Or have you ever read a sentence and by the end, you have forgotten what you read at the beginning? Let's face it – probably quite a few sentences in this book. These are examples of how working memory works (or doesn't).

Working memory is a crucial brain skill that enables us to hold and manipulate information in our minds over extremely short periods of time. It is a little bit like having a mental notepad in which the brain scribbles information for a few seconds, to use it for a quick task. It might not even be important enough to process into regular short-term memory. This mental notepad temporarily stores information we need for tasks such as learning, reasoning and comprehension.

You might see some psychologists include all short-term memory in their description of working memory. This inconsistency in terminology is a bit frustrating and makes it extremely difficult to read the research papers sometimes. Most scientists now separate short-term memory (memory over hours and even a few days) from the 'scribble-pad' (extremely short working memory of a few seconds or minutes).

If we think of working memory as the ability to keep a few items in our head while we do the shopping, for example, even this involves several different brain processes. These processes include directing your attention to the items you want to remember and coordinating your brain activities.

We need a working memory for words and sounds as well as objects and abstract thoughts, so this also involves processing verbal (and/or written) information or using a 'visuospatial sketchpad', which handles how we process our physical surroundings and how we picture things in our minds. Trying to remember that phone number someone read out to you is a good example of verbal and auditory working memory, while forgetting where you put your mobile phone ten seconds ago is an example of a lack of 'visuospatial' working memory.

If you have problems with working memory, it can make seemingly simple things very complicated. If your boss says to you, 'I need you to do three things for me,' and you don't have a pen and paper to hand, the chances are you might not remember any or all of those three things. Far less importantly, it might mean making a cup of tea is challenging, as you have to remember that you boiled the kettle. James usually takes about seven attempts to make a cup of tea. Then forgets to drink it.

In general, adults with ADHD have a similar range of long-term and 'normal' short-term memory. Some of us are good; some not so good. On the other hand, we often have a worse working memory than a typical person. This appears to be because we struggle with both storage and retrieval of very short-term information, resulting in a failure in recalling relevant facts.[70]

On a day-to-day basis, having poor working memory can result in forgotten appointments, misplaced items or difficulty following a complex recipe. Put bluntly, it is a bloody nightmare. When poor working memory is combined with distractibility, it means we can easily go on 'side quests',

EXECUTIVE FUNCTIONS AND ADHD

quickly forgetting whichever task we intended to focus on and instead ending up doing something else, sometimes for hours.

Inhibitory control

Someone once said that ADHD is like having a Ferrari body with bicycle brakes. The Ferrari represents hyperactivity of the body and mind rather than a brain that is actually faster, unfortunately. But the brake comparison is very accurate. ADHD often feels as if we are less able to put the brakes on our thoughts or our actions. These brakes are called inhibitory control.

Inhibitory control is the ability to override an instinctive response in favour of something more appropriate. 'I won't eat all of those cakes because I will get ill,' for example. Having these brakes in our brain is crucial for both basic tasks in life, such as resisting the temptation to eat a full pack of biscuits, as well as the more complex social interactions, such as choosing not to express every thought in a conversation with someone we have just met. Inhibitory control is an executive function that enables us to pause and think before acting and also to choose our responses to align with social norms and expectations. This is often described as the ability to have 'free will' rather than just responding to everything automatically.

Poor inhibitory control can manifest in many ways and can significantly affect our personal, academic and professional lives. Some of the most common challenges adults with

ADHD face is the tendency to interrupt conversations (or always wanting to) and struggling to wait until it is the right time to interject (or not to interject at all). It is very common for people with ADHD to speak or answer a question without having fully thought about it, which can lead to a lot of shame and self-chastisement.

We get that feeling of reward from impulsively sharing our immediate thoughts and responses and, at the same time, avoid the problem of forgetting what we wanted to say if our working memory is also a bit poor. Interrupting a lot is similar to another common example of lacking inhibitory control, which is making impulse purchases. The immediate reward of buying something, even if it isn't needed, often overshadows the long-term goal (of saving money, for example), resulting in high levels of personal debt. Impulse spending is the reason why James purchased six guitars during lockdown, and then gave three away, before buying two more. We should add – without playing ANY of them.

More seriously, poor inhibitory control can also lead to engaging in risky behaviours, such as reckless driving, substance abuse or 'risky sexual behaviour', which was covered in Chapter 9. The immediate thrill or perceived benefit can outweigh the consideration of any potential long-term harm. The impulsiveness that comes from poor inhibitory control means it is the only real executive function that is part of the main diagnosis pathway of ADHD, as it is part of the 'hyperactivity/impulsivity' presentation of around two-thirds of adults with ADHD. But it isn't the only one we struggle with.

EXECUTIVE FUNCTIONS AND ADHD

Cognitive flexibility

Ironically, considering how often we are told this is an ADHD skill, cognitive inflexibility could be described as 'problems thinking outside the box'. If you drive the same way to work every day for ten years, but one day you give a colleague a lift and they point out a faster, shorter route, even if they are correct, this can be startling and challenging for people with ADHD. This is an example of a lack of cognitive flexibility: 'I always take that route!'

Cognitive flexibility means changing the thought processes you are having. This is another crucial element of being human and is an executive function that enables you to adapt both your thoughts and behaviour in response to changing circumstances, demands or perspectives. It includes the ability to switch between different tasks, or to accept change that someone else imposes on you. It also enables you to think about, and assess, more than one concept at the same time.

Cognitive flexibility is a really essential skill at the very heart of problem-solving, learning and creativity. We will come back to ADHD and creativity later! This mental flexibility also enables us to update our understanding of any situation based on new information, to adjust our approach when a situation changes, and to view problems from various angles. The world around us changes constantly, and being adaptable is essential to progress.

In general, people with ADHD are less 'cognitively flexible' than people in the general population. This is probably because the areas of the brain needed to adapt to change are less active in ADHD people.[71] This concept can be a challenging thing to accept, and it definitely doesn't mean we are stupid or lacking intelligence or even creativity. It means that we will sometimes persevere with the wrong approach to a problem that is repeatedly not working, whereas most people would be more able to stop, take a breath and think for a second. If you have ever repeatedly failed at a problem but your brain refused to stop and try something new, you might recognise how challenges with cognitive flexibility can make our lives rather frustrating.

Emotional and cognitive decision-making

Oddly enough, although emotional dysregulation is an issue for most adults with ADHD, we are often also better at making emotional decisions than purely cognitive (or logical and emotionless) ones. Sadly, we aren't necessarily better than everyone else. That was nearly a superpower. The ability to make 'emotional' choices is known as 'affective decision-making' (where 'affective' is a scientific term for 'emotional' or 'based on mood'). Both cognitive and affective decision-making are crucial aspects of executive function. This is how someone makes choices based on either intellectual or emotional outcomes and preferences. These processes are complex, involving the integration of thoughts and emotional responses, evaluation of potential outcomes, and the regulation of impulsive tendencies.

EXECUTIVE FUNCTIONS AND ADHD

Time management

The perception of time and time management are crucial for effective functioning in everyday life. Time management is a cognitive ability that involves planning, organising and effectively using time to achieve goals. Part of this ability requires the brain to be able to perceive the passing of time.

While no single brain region has been identified as responsible for time perception, the front parts of the brain and the imaginatively named 'time cells', found in a part of the brain called the hippocampus, are thought to be heavily involved.[72] These 'time cells' fire electrical signals at successive moments as time passes and we experience the world around us. What is very apparent to anyone with ADHD is that these cells don't work in the same way in our brains, leading to something that is sometimes referred to informally as 'time blindness'.

While people with ADHD are of course not totally blind to time, they often struggle with two key areas of time management: time estimation and time.[73] To some extent, even seeing time as a linear thing where there is a future version of us is problematic, so maybe three areas.

Time estimation refers to two related skills: the ability to estimate how much time has passed without using a watch or a timer, and the ability to estimate how long it will take to complete a task or activity in the future.[74] Now, depending on the occasion, people may feel that time passes quickly or slowly. A good example of people feeling time is passing

209

slowly would be the experience of anyone who has ever seen James speak publicly about ADHD. Multiple studies have shown, however, that people with ADHD commonly under- or over-estimate how much time has passed, and this can include time intervals from seconds to minutes as well as hours, days and years.[75]

Time reproduction is the ability to reproduce a specific duration of time. Let's say you watch someone turn a light switch on for a while, then off again, and then you try to match the time they left the light on. Almost all studies looking into time reproduction show that guessing at this time period is impaired in people with ADHD.[76]

Risky decisions

People with ADHD generally engage in more risk-taking on a day-to-day basis than people without ADHD.[77] It may seem odd to circle back to decision-making, but one particular form of decision-making is very relevant in ADHD: decisions where risk is involved. If you are someone with ADHD that seems risk-averse (such as Alex), this is because ADHD can be a challenge with 'risk perception' as well as risky decision-making. If you can't tell what is risky, this could lead to a fear of ever taking a risk, but more often and more damagingly with ADHD, it can lead to some quite risky choices.

As we have mentioned throughout the book, adults with ADHD are on average more likely to have accidents, drive unsafely, engage in risky sexual behaviour and struggle

EXECUTIVE FUNCTIONS AND ADHD

with substance use. This suggests that people with ADHD may be more likely to make risky decisions. Despite this seemingly obvious link, until recently there hasn't been a great deal of research into this.

Part of this 'risky decision-making' is due to that fact that people with ADHD often have altered reward sensitivity, which can contribute to risk-taking by emphasising potential gains while ignoring possible losses. Add a dash of impulsivity to our natural aversion to delayed reward and this can lead to dismissing wiser alternatives. With behavioural disinhibition that can make a recipe for risky decisions.

Although the 'real world' examples, such as increased accidents and unsafe sex in the ADHD population, might make it seem obvious that poor risk perception and risky decisions are to blame, researchers often have to get into a controlled environment, such as a laboratory, to study and really understand something. Or pretend to, which James successfully did for almost twenty years as a laboratory scientist.

For risky decisions, a research study often takes the form of a mock gambling exercise. While some studies disagree, a large study published in 2016 gathered lots of data from smaller studies together and found that, yes, people with ADHD are more likely to take risks in a controlled environment.[78] The authors of that study suggested that reduced risk aversion and overt risk-seeking may be to blame. Whatever the biological or psychological cause, it is clear that our perception of risk, and the decisions we make based on this perception, can be flawed.

SUMMARY

Executive functions describe the more 'evolved' or higher-order thinking skills such as organisation, prioritisation and working memory that humans use to navigate life and all its complexities. ADHD is strongly associated with impairments in executive functions, and this can significantly affect daily life, including educational or work challenges, social interactions, self-care and general health and well-being.

Understanding that struggling with these impairments can help people with ADHD better understand and accept themselves, and in the right environment and with the right support, lacking normal executive functions doesn't have to be a barrier to success or happiness. One of the key areas in which executive function challenges really affect us is in trying to build connections with people and maintain trust and support. In the next chapter, we will look more broadly at the effect of ADHD on relationships, with romantic partners as well as at work and with family and friends.

CHAPTER 13

Sex, relationships and ADHD

Around a third of all marriages end in divorce, so relationships can be complex for anyone. When you add at least one neurospicy person, it can become far more difficult to navigate the natural ups and downs of any relationship.[79] FYI: we are still not sure about the term 'neurospicy'.

This difficulty is true of relationships with family members, friends and work colleagues, as well as romantic relationships, and is probably not that surprising if you think about how all of the challenges of ADHD that we have discussed in this book could affect a relationship. These could include the adult with ADHD not paying attention to someone, forgetfulness, regulating emotions, accepting rejection or criticism, making decisions ... the list goes on.

Any of those ADHD issues individually would make managing or maintaining relationships more difficult, whether this is with people in your family, at work or your friendship group but especially (if you are lucky enough to have one) your partner (or partners – we are very modern like that). Now when you combine many of those ADHD traits, the whole relationship thing can become a minefield that needs serious communication and empathy from both sides to stay healthy.

There are many examples and experiences where the behaviours and traits of adults with ADHD have led to friction in relationships. This isn't the same as blame and is a question of interpretation and communication. We have all experienced these frictions and will continue to do so. The ADHD isn't going anywhere. Examples of this could include not always listening effectively to a partner when they are speaking to us, forgetting to send a birthday card (or even a text) to a good friend, or missing a work meeting because you put it in your calendar at the wrong time. Adults with ADHD do this sort of thing on a daily basis, but how this is interpreted by the other person and how this is explained by us is absolutely crucial for a healthy relationship. If both parties understand the reasons behind those scenarios above, it starts to make sense that this is a result of ADHD, rather than of someone who doesn't care about the people in their life.

Not listening to a partner when they are speaking to you can be difficult because of mind wandering and attention issues. Even when we really want to listen to that person, it isn't always possible. Forgetting to send a friend that birthday card, or to be honest forgetting they exist at all (friends, not birthday cards), is quite common because many adults with ADHD have what we unscientifically call 'object invisibility' or 'object impermanence'. What this means is that

214

SEX, RELATIONSHIPS AND ADHD

if a thing or a person isn't very 'visible' to someone with ADHD, that thing (or person) can temporarily cease to exist in our mind. Or it certainly feels that way (they probably do continue to exist out there somewhere).

This is like having a Post-it™ note on your computer screen with the words 'Call Susan'. This note has been there for three years — it blends into the background until we almost literally don't 'see it' even when looking directly at it. Psychologists say that true object impermanence is only seen in very young babies who, for example, wouldn't know that shiny keys exist if you hide them behind your back. The prevailing view seems to be that adults don't actually think that something 'out of sight, out of mind' doesn't exist, but we think ADHD very much feels like this sometimes — 'object impermanence' is a useful term to describe it.

The perception that we might not care about other people if we miss meetings, for example, because we might have put it in our diary on the wrong date, at the wrong time or place or not added it to a diary at all, is also quite damaging unless this is communicated properly. In reality, this also comes down to classic ADHD challenges of executive function, such as organisation: that so-called time blindness and working memory. This is the reason why it once took James five attempts to book a blood pressure test at his local doctors' surgery, because he kept getting the day and time wrong. Alex has a rule that if he is told the time of any appointment it MUST go in his calendar at that moment or it never will. The optimism of thinking we will remember it later is rarely accurate.

It is also important at this point to state that it is OK if you are that partner, friend or business colleague to feel put out by this. We are not asking people to be fine with things that affect them negatively. Of course, some of the ways in which ADHD impacts our behaviour does affect other people, even though that isn't our intention. ADHD is a *reason* and not an *excuse,* but we are asking for some understanding and a conversation about why that happens and what we can do to reduce it.

The important thing to agree is that in any relationship involving at least one person with ADHD, the feelings and needs of everybody in that relationship are valid and should be respected. Where things often become difficult is when somebody in a relationship struggles to accept that ADHD is a reason for these things. This is true if the person with ADHD is the one who hasn't emotionally accepted their own condition, or if the other person doesn't have ADHD and won't accept or doesn't understand the ADHD diagnosis. In this last scenario, this can lead to people interpreting ADHD behaviours as their partner not being interested in them or their friend being inconsiderate / not caring about them.

Similarly, at work, people might unfairly decide that ADHD traits mean their work colleague is a bit of a flake. Language around ADHD often includes terms such as this. James was once told by an employer (who thought this was fine): 'We know you're a flake, but you're our flake.' This is not fine.

From the perspective of adults with ADHD, a big challenge is to ask for help and support to reduce the chances of these mistakes (or their impact). This can often feel quite difficult or embarrassing to admit at work, as most people appear to handle seemingly simple admin with few problems at all.

There are countless different effects of ADHD and approaches to handling them depending on the nature of the relationship. In no particular order, we will cover issues with these relationships for the rest of this chapter.

Friendships

Most of the evidence about friendships and ADHD comes from studies of children, teenagers or university students. Either this is because adults don't have friends, or more likely it is because there are glaring holes in research on adult ADHD and friendships. As usual, it is worth reiterating that not all research is good. The findings of any study are only as good as the design of that study, and (for many reasons, but usually financial) many studies in ADHD are poorly designed or not very conclusive. This is probably one of the reasons why there are oddly conflicting findings when you look at ADHD in friendships. One very small study, for example, found that increased ADHD symptoms led to stronger same-sex friendships,[80] but a much better study reported that children and young adults with ADHD had significantly fewer friends, lower quality friendships and poorer friendship interactions.[81]

The broad consensus is that people with ADHD generally struggle to foster or maintain long-lasting friendships (and from our lived experience, we would also recognise this problem, although James can't seem to shake off

Alex despite quite a lot of effort). There are many possible reasons for this: the stigma associated with ADHD, the way in which adults with ADHD often forget to stay in touch or struggle to control emotions, social phobia (which is found in as many as 49.5 per cent of people with ADHD[82]) and partly because, to be honest, it can sometimes be really hard being the friend of somebody with ADHD!

It is particularly unfair that adults with ADHD can struggle with friendships, given how valuable they can be. Having a close friend who can provide non-judgmental support has been shown to assist ADHDers with engaging in social activities.[83] Because it is common for us to experience social isolation, it isn't surprising that adults with ADHD often seek support groups, including online support groups. In fact, people with ADHD have been shown to have higher social media use than the general population (possibly for other reasons around the need for external validation as well).

Support groups are invaluable to many of us, but these are not the same as friendships in the traditional sense, often (not always) lacking the day-to-day support and camaraderie that one-to-one friendship can bring (or so we have been told). These more intimate friendships can be difficult when you have ADHD. ADHD also makes it harder to stay on top of friendships (not literally). With time blindness and motivational challenges, it is very easy to lose track of how long it has been since you have seen someone, or to remember to call a friend when you said you would. Even answering a text message can be challenging on some days – and don't get us started on voicemails.

Tip for contacting your ADHD friends: ask before sending voice messages! For both of us, listening to any voice message for longer than three seconds is torture. All of this can make friends think you don't care about them enough, especially if they don't understand or accept the challenges of ADHD.

Family relationships

At the risk of sounding like a stuck record, the research into ADHD and family relationships also isn't great. Despite this, there is some evidence that issues can arise between siblings (and with other family members too) where one or both of them has ADHD. Studies have shown that when one person in the family has ADHD, it can affect how positively their parents, siblings and other family members feel about their own everyday life. One study even found that siblings felt victimised by their ADHD sibling and that this victimisation was often overlooked in the family.[84]

What often complicates familial relationships is the fact that due to the genetic component of ADHD, there is usually more than one member of the family with ADHD, diagnosed or not. If, as evidence suggests, first-degree relatives of somebody with ADHD are between five and seven times more likely to also have ADHD,[85] managing relationships within a family group when multiple people have ADHD adds a layer of complexity. Especially if they don't know it or don't have access to support. This complexity comes in several forms. Firstly, there is some evidence that 'ADHD families' *may* function differently,[86] with parents of ADHD children tending to use criticism more, and affection less.[87] This may not be 'because' of ADHD itself, but rather 'because of growing up without support for ADHD'. Spending your formative years in an environment like this can build up dysfunctional familial relationships.

Secondly, disclosing ADHD to family members can cause friction as family members may not want to consider or believe that ADHD is real, or that they may also have it. This is anecdotally often the case with parents, as the stigma of 'ADHD being caused by bad parenting' is very much ingrained in society (despite being a myth!).

Workplace relationships

The chances are that if you work for an employer with more than forty employees, you work with at least one person with ADHD. You may not know it, they may not know it, but with an estimated incidence of 2.5–5 per cent, most of us work with someone who has ADHD, and they are probably undiagnosed. Chapter 14 includes more information on navigating ADHD and careers/workplace, but for people trying to understand the effect on work relationships, ADHD has been associated with disruptive behaviour, job performance problems and risk-taking in the workplace.[88]

Some of the other common and persistent issues faced by adults with ADHD professionally include missing social cues and expected norms, interrupting or talking over other people and being less able to regulate emotional responses leading to quick tempers or visible frustration.

SEX, RELATIONSHIPS AND ADHD

This often leads to the attribution of labels including 'unreliable', 'emotional' and 'difficult to work with' – and these labels are hard to shake. As a result of this, ADHD adults often mask in the workplace, trying to fit in and look 'normal', very often at a high cost to both mental and physical health. In many cases, this masking is NOT because our behaviour is disruptive, harmful or wrong. In fact, many of the typical expectations of behaviour are simply different, rather than better or worse. Despite this, we as a society tend to treat the majority option as the 'correct' way of doing things.[89] This is called normative discrimination, and it is very frustrating.

If, for example, you are the colleague of somebody with ADHD, who occasionally drops the ball or overreacts, you may respond negatively to this or find it frustrating yourself. However, with an understanding of ADHD comes a better understanding of why these things happen. The colleague who doesn't reply to emails quickly, the employee who is often late or who (from your perspective) seems to drift off when you are in a meeting with them. These behaviours can irritate some people, and that irritation can make for hostile workplace relationships. While there is legislation to protect employees in the workplace (in the UK, this is the 2010 Equality Act), ADHD symptoms can not only impair the ability of an employee to work productively under typical social expectations, but they can also cause friction with colleagues lacking the contextual knowledge of ADHD. More importantly, it is often because the process that works for most people needs to be tweaked slightly for adults with ADHD. For example, we often struggle to reply to emails with a question buried at the end of a long, pointless paragraph of unrelated information. And more than one question is also a challenge. Short, clear requests in a separate email are far more helpful and don't cost anything more than some thought in advance.

Romantic relationships

It is very important to start this section with two facts. Firstly, almost all research into romantic relationships has been conducted in cisgendered, heteronormative couples. This really needs to change, as there is a massive gap in our understanding of ADHD. Secondly, and before we get too morose about something as wonderful as romantic relationships, it is important to state that many adults with ADHD have happy, fulfilling and successful romantic relationships. If you are one of these people, then chapeaux. It is likely that your happiness, fulfilment and success come from good communication and a sense of teamwork in your relationship. There can be lots of positives in having a romantic partner with ADHD. We can sometimes hyperfocus on romance or sex, our impulsive actions can be romantic or endearing … Erm, that is about it.

Romantic relationships in general – and particularly in modern times – can be complicated, but almost universally the evidence around relationships where at least one person has ADHD suggests that 'relationshipping' with ADHD is even more complicated. This information is widely discussed and has even reached the glossy magazines.[90] We are also not sure about the word 'relationshipping'. Regardless, romantic relationships are likely to be the

SEX, RELATIONSHIPS AND ADHD

hardest of all relationship types to manage with ADHD successfully.

Even if you are not in a relationship, being comfortable with being single or with dating can be challenging with ADHD. The fear of rejection can lead to avoiding romance entirely and can lead to long periods in the sexual wilderness (also known as 'James's twenties'). Unlike James in his twenties, young adult heterosexual men with ADHD are more likely to have lifetime romantic partners than men without ADHD, whereas young adult heterosexual women with ADHD reported having fewer lifetime romantic relationships than reported by women without ADHD. We imagine that this reflects some of the stigma around being a woman with ADHD, but we don't know exactly why this is.

Interestingly, young men with the predominantly inattentive type of ADHD (formerly ADD) seem to be slower to reach typical dating milestones, such as their first serious dating partner, than people with combined type ADHD or young men without ADHD. Clearly, many ADHD issues can impact dating, but fortunately, 'never being impulsive' is unlikely to be one of them.

The core symptoms of both inattention and hyperactivity/impulsivity are enough to cause relationship problems, but add in generous helpings of rejection sensitivity and a sprinkle of emotional dysregulation (covered in Chapter 11) and there are a thousand different recipes in which ADHD can cause tensions in any relationship. It has been estimated that up to 96 per cent of spouses of adults with ADHD reported that their ADHD partner's symptoms made household management more difficult.[91]

ADHD partners often struggle with organisation or may be more likely to lose important items (such as passports). We may have issues with impulse spending or may not be able to contribute as much towards shared domestic chores to the satisfaction of our partner. All of this can be frustrating and, while we completely understand that feeling, we would remind anyone that this isn't a question of laziness or willpower. We want to do those things more than anyone else wants us to be able to do them. The frustration of struggling with these simple tasks is a fundamental basis for some of the self-esteem issues we face as a community. These frictions can then ultimately lead to the partners of people with ADHD feeling as if they have to parent their partner, which can impact intimacy.

As difficult as it is, we must also talk about some of the negative outcomes of relationships in this section, including infidelity, divorce and intimate partner violence. There is strong evidence that, *on average*, relationships where one or more adults have ADHD are more likely to see risky sexual behaviour and infidelity, end in separation or divorce or be *either* the victim *or* perpetrator of intimate partner violence. One of the most important parts in that last sentence is 'on average'. Having ADHD doesn't mean you *will* be in one of these relationships or face relationship challenges at all. The first of these issues – showing (or acting on) interest in people outside a relationship – is easy to understand when you consider the impulsivity, poor risk perception and 'dopamine seeking' that many adults with ADHD have. A survey of over 3,000 people with ADHD by Ari Tuckman for his book, *ADHD After Dark*, found that around 40 per cent of both men and women with ADHD had at least one physical affair and nearly 50 per cent of women (and 43 per cent of men) had at least one emotional affair at some point in their life.

Within romantic relationships, we also face specific challenges with the thorny issue of intimacy, including physical intimacy and sex. Not literally thorny – usually. And, of course, not everyone is in a relationship, but in what we only assume is a very modern twist, *sex still happens whether in a relationship or not!*

Intimacy and sex

To quote the band Suede (James insisted) – sex: it is simple and complex. The statement is both accurate and enduring. Healthy and loving romantic relationships are usually an important part of life in adulthood, and often the success of a romantic relationship relies on intimacy. Intimacy in romantic relationships isn't just about sex; it refers to the deep emotional, psychological and physical closeness between two people (or more – we like to think we are modern, open-minded authors).

Intimacy is a vital component of healthy, fulfilling relationships and can take many forms: emotional intimacy, intellectual intimacy, trust and vulnerability and physical intimacy, among others. It is important to point out that there is probably no more difficult subject to talk about when it comes to ADHD and relationships, so there may be some material here that you might find personally difficult to read but we felt needed to be included.

Relationships in which at least one adult has ADHD may experience a range of challenges related to intimacy, sexual health and activity. Again, not all relationships with adults with ADHD will have these issues, and experiences can vary widely. Once again, the variability within the ADHD community means we are not all the same: the impact of one person's ADHD response can lead to diametrically opposing behaviours and this is certainly the case when it comes to sex.

Adults with ADHD may have little to no interest in sex at all (possibly due to RSD), they might be hypersexual, or they could be somewhere in the middle. (Not literally. Sometimes literally). We may masturbate more or less than average. We may have sensory issues that mean some sex acts are either overwhelming or feel completely pointless due to the variability in our sensory thresholds.

Issues such as distractibility and mind wandering mean that even during sex it is quite common for our attention to suddenly switch to, say, a cobweb that is hanging from the ceiling. Maintaining a state of arousal while at the same time thinking, 'When was the last time I vacuumed the cobwebs?' is difficult. Not impossible, but difficult and VERY hard to explain to your partner. Whether it is distractibility, impulsivity, emotional regulation or rejection sensitivity leading to poor communication and self-esteem issues, you name it, if it is an ADHD-related trait, it can probably have an impact on our sex life.

SEX, RELATIONSHIPS AND ADHD

A fascinating anonymous survey on ADHD and sex was published in 2023.[92] Among the many notable statistics was the observation that adults with ADHD (both males and females) had a higher preference for same-sex or either-sex partners as well as higher rates of 'sexting' and masturbation. We were also more likely to contract sexually transmitted infections (please remember these survey results aren't saying all of us face these issues, just the statistics are higher). This survey also reported that adults with ADHD were more likely to be sexually adventurous and less satisfied with their partners. The levels and range of sexual interests differed between the sexes, but women acted on them more commonly than men.

Feeling unhappy with issues around intimacy and sex is such a common problem, and it is important for people with ADHD to know that help is available. Seeking support from sex/couples counsellors to strengthen a relationship isn't a sign of weakness. It is a sign of strength and respect. Learning strategies to address the challenges that ADHD brings to a relationship can be fun and innovative and will even increase the chances of relationship success.

Partners of adults with ADHD can also benefit from education and support to better understand and navigate these issues together. With the right communication and strategies, adults with ADHD can have healthy and fulfilling romantic relationships.

SUMMARY

Whether the relationships are platonic, professional or intimate, the core challenges of ADHD could be seen as a list of obstacles for both making and maintaining connections with people. From inattention at work and home, to feelings of restlessness and impulsive actions, clearly both parties in an ADHD relationship have to communicate how this affects them and what they can do to work together for a healthy future.

While there are many coping strategies and treatments for these ADHD traits and behaviours, the most important factor for relationships and ADHD is healthy communication. Clearly expressing our challenges and expectations, planning achievable goals and tasks together as a team and safely discussing the effects of ADHD on both members of a relationship will help everyone involved. It isn't always as easy as it sounds but it is always good to talk about it.

This communication is also key for getting tasks done in a relationship, at work or anywhere else in life. In the next chapter, we will explore the reasons and some solutions to getting started with jobs, seeing them through and getting them fully finished. Alliteration works better though, so we will call it prioritisation, procrastination, perfectionism and productivity.

CHAPTER 14

ADHD & the 4 Ps: prioritisation, procrastination, perfectionism and productivity

Of all the issues that ADHD causes, engaging with tasks that *we want to engage with* is probably one of the most frustrating. People often wrongly assume that we never want to do those tasks or we are being dishonest when we say we are planning to do them. The reality is that we can often struggle, even if we do want to be productive and genuinely intend to get those tasks done.

Dr Russell Barkley, the godfather of ADHD research, sometimes calls ADHD 'Intention Deficit Disorder' because there is a gap between what we intend to do and our actions (known as the intention-action gap). For example, we may fully intend to pay our tax bill, but when we go to fill in the forms, something stops us and that simple task can suddenly feel incredibly overwhelming.

The simple act of logging onto the computer or opening that bill in the first place can feel impossibly hard. So we hide from it. Or we put it off. We do this for many reasons, but usually people struggle with completing tasks due to issues with prioritisation, procrastination or perfectionism.

In this chapter, we will discuss how issues with prioritisation, procrastination and perfectionism are far more common in adults with ADHD than in the general population. We will explain their impact on productivity and discuss what we can do to start addressing those challenges in line with our ADHD.

Prioritisation

Pretty much everybody with ADHD has been asked at some point, 'Have you tried a planner? What about a to-do list?' This is one of the first things most people suggest to us in the workplace. The answer? Yes. Yes, we have. The challenge is figuring out the *type* of planning that works for us. Repeatedly buying many pretty notebooks and a nice pen works for some of us (Alex), but definitely not for others (James). One of the reasons is based on personality and preference, because we are all different. Another reason depends on the kind of ADHD challenges we have and the tasks we need to plan (which are also all different). There is no single answer for all of us.

If you think about your typical day, there are probably several tasks or activities that you could choose to focus on first, especially if you had that to-do list in front of you. Choosing exactly which tasks or activities to start with requires the ability to prioritise. You can do this right now if you have a to-do list in front of you. Have a look at it. Does it seem overwhelming? Does it seem as if every task looks equally important? Many adults with ADHD struggle to figure out the order in which to do things and where to begin in the first place. It isn't as simple as 'do them in order of priority' if you don't know how to choose the priority.

If you are thinking, 'Hang on, I am able to prioritise well' (as Alex used to think), this is fantastic. That could be because we don't all have the same deficits, and no one can tell you how your ADHD manifests. BUT it could also be that we sometimes don't realise that we have prioritised things that don't necessarily help the overall goal. For example, we might do things that benefit other people over our own needs and preferences (James), or we might choose priorities that make us look good in front of other people (Alex). If it helps, we can call that last one external motivation instead of showing off.

According to some evidence (and certainly in our experience with the community), adults with ADHD tend to give a higher priority not only to things that have an imminent deadline but also to tasks that might be seen by or benefit other people.[93] This may be because ADHD is associated with a lack of internal motivation. Internal motivation is the desire to engage in an activity because it is enjoyable or rewarding, and this can be influenced by lots of factors, including our needs, desires, goals and values. If we struggle with a sense of self and with self-esteem, for example, we might tend to prioritise others' needs first. If we tend to struggle with internal motivation, it is probably no surprise when we prioritise things that are going to be visible to other people.

This means that adults with ADHD are more likely to rely on external motivation to get things done. External motivation is the drive to engage in an activity because of external rewards, such as making someone happy or receiving praise or attention. This has a direct impact on prioritisation, as it makes it significantly more likely that adults with ADHD will prioritise tasks and activities that are for the benefit (or awareness) of other people, and not necessarily because that activity is the best choice at that moment to achieve a specific goal.

This issue with low internal motivation is so common in ADHD because it is directly related to how the reward centre in the brain works (or doesn't work), which we talked about in Chapter 10. If that isn't enough, we are also more likely to assign importance to other people due to RSD, imposter syndrome and low self-esteem.

Prioritising is such an important ability, particularly in the workplace, so it might be useful to look at how your prioritisation skills can be improved. How we prioritise things usually depends on two connected factors. The first requires that we plan our priorities effectively using several of those pesky executive functions, which are covered in Chapter 12. Examples of these might include a mental comprehension of what the task is, thinking about how urgent the task is (and how long it takes) as well as understanding what needs to be done to accomplish it and why we should even do it in the first place.

These are all executive function issues that include logical planning as well as our emotions. It is important to try and be aware of our emotions, because prioritisation can be affected by factors such as fear of failure, impostor syndrome, boredom, anger, fear of being told off, people-pleasing (often due to rejection sensitivity) and many more.

When trying to engage with any task, our brain will try to call up memories about this type of task from a previous experience (or a similar one to compare it to). For example, if we were building a bonfire at a campsite, we might prioritise looking for dry wood in places where we have found dry wood before, such as underneath trees? (We should have asked Bear Grylls). This seems like a logical plan for building a fire, but the emotions that accompany those old memories contribute to how we rate the significance of the task, as well as how much it interests us and whether negative experiences in the past have left emotional scars that can block us from doing that task. So, if we once made a bonfire but it was raining and the wood was wet, we might prioritise looking for dry wood first. But if we once got bitten by a hedgehog while making that bonfire, we might prioritise buying gloves or not building a bonfire in the first place as it is far too dangerous (note: we don't know if hedgehogs bite). Transfer that to the workplace, and seemingly simple non-bonfire-related tasks can have very different emotional associations that stop us from acting.

We have already discussed that ADHD means we are more likely to prioritise based on external motivation. But it also means that we are often unable to transfer past events well or just find the idea of writing everything down too tedious, so struggle to make a strong priority list at all. Without developing some system of prioritisation to make up for the issues caused by ADHD, we often either do nothing (task paralysis) or default to tasks that are imminent or overdue (displacement tasks).

Fortunately, some approaches that can be used for prioritisation (in theory but definitely not always) can help us decide what needs to be tackled first and how to start. To plan any task at all, it is useful to use something like S.M.A.R.T goals (explained more in Chapter 16). These can help with prioritisation as well as the other elements of productivity in this chapter. There are generally four things to consider when trying to prioritise: urgency, importance, difficulty and well-being. Let's explore these.

Urgency

Urgent activities are usually (but not always) associated with achieving our (or someone else's) goals. Something is usually considered urgent because we have been given a deadline (even by ourselves), such as a bill that needs to be paid or a project at work that is due. Adults with ADHD are even more inclined than everyone else to work 'hyperbolically'. In this case, that doesn't mean working in an exaggerated way. It means that the amount of engagement in a task increases more and more the closer we get to a deadline (the shape of a hyperbolic curve – Google it to know what it looks like).

You might recognise that you need to feel as if there is a crisis, some urgency or a pressing deadline that determines what has to be done and provides the motivation to do it (sometimes). These 'urgent' tasks are often the ones we concentrate on. They demand attention because the consequences of not dealing with them are immediate and possibly negative in terms of how other people view us. In other words, they are close enough to now and powerful enough that we can more easily 'feel' the potential consequence of failure.

Importance

The second factor of importance is a tricky one. Importance *should* be about you! Will this task help with your personal or professional development? Will it help you achieve a goal that you want to achieve? Because these questions are based around doing something for ourselves, it is easy to see why this is a difficult factor to use in prioritisation with ADHD, because the low self-esteem that we commonly have often means we don't value ourselves enough to do tasks that are *for* us. Having a set of clear values written down can help with understanding how 'important' a task is because we often ignore that objective list in favour of something that happens to be right there, right now.

Difficulty

This is an example of how ADHD can require a different approach to the way the rest of the world works (or thinks it works) most efficiently. With some people with ADHD (including both of us), it sometimes helps to start the day with a task that is 'low-hanging fruit'. By picking an easy win, and trying to complete it, we can give ourselves a little 'bump of dopamine' because we have achieved something (we know it isn't really just dopamine). This achievement can then be used to kickstart our day, so we might tackle other more difficult tasks. You might have heard that many people do the exact opposite. This is sometimes called 'eat the frog first',[94] where if you do the most difficult thing at the start, the rest of a task is easier. Of course, this might work for some adults with ADHD, but in our experience, this is a classic example of strategies that aren't designed for the neurodivergent ADHD community.

It is true that the science says that not starting with a 'difficult task' might affect self-worth (because it is looming over us) but with ADHD, everything looms over us except that one weird hyperfocus. Seemingly simple tasks can be cripplingly difficult, and self-esteem and self-worth are already seriously affected. So if you try the low-hanging fruit approach and it works, don't feel you have to eat the frog first because that's what other people do. Make sure you work within your ADHD preferences.

Well-being

Finally, we have well-being. You can't judge the value of a task unless you are sure what success looks like and how healthy it will be to complete it. Something that has been achieved but at a terrible cost is called a 'Pyrrhic victory' – this is a common challenge for the ADHD community. We think it is vital to include a measure of personal success and wellbeing to any priority list. We would suggest that when you are building a task list to get something done, it is important to include questions such as these:

1. Is that task or activity something that will make you feel better about yourself?

2. If it is, it should be a higher priority. Is it something you tend to do well?

3. Is it something you tend to enjoy doing?

It is important to work within your personal preferences but again, you can probably see the inherent flaw in this approach because most people with ADHD tend to describe themselves as people-pleasers or struggle to find the motivation to do things solely for themselves.

It is very difficult to explain to people without ADHD how difficult it is to prioritise sometimes. People with ADHD just tend to 'do stuff' and are usually more able to identify what is a priority and then engage with it. Having problems with prioritisation can lead to issues in relationships (especially if we don't prioritise our partner's needs or expectations with tasks around the house, for example). It can also lead to significant issues in the workplace, as we tend to 'firefight' – deal with whatever is imminent because we didn't deal with it when it first came to light. This leads us nicely onto the topic of procrastination.

Procrastination

One of the diagnostic symptoms of ADHD is 'Often avoids, dislikes, or is reluctant to do tasks that require mental effort over a long period of time.'[95] This symptom almost exactly matches the definition of procrastination. Despite the link between ADHD and procrastination being almost universally recognised, there is surprisingly little research on the subject. What research there is reports that ADHD symptoms positively correlate with procrastination[96] and 'task aversiveness', meaning the more symptoms of ADHD one has, the more likely you are to avoid or delay engagement in tasks.[97]

Procrastination is a failure of self-regulation that means failing to start or complete tasks that are known to be important, even though delaying them will have negative consequences.[98] Procrastination can take two forms. Active procrastinators tend to prefer to work under pressure, effectively choosing to procrastinate, whereas 'passive' procrastinators fit the traditional image of procrastination: an inability to engage with a task, leading to problems completing tasks on time. Although the second is a classic ADHD trait, there is some evidence that both types are linked to ADHD symptoms.[99] In other words, we don't always mean to procrastinate but sometimes we do it on purpose. Why is this?

Firstly, we must come back to reward. Tasks that we don't find emotionally rewarding are usually more difficult to engage with (as we have touched on earlier in the book). This is because of the way the reward centre of the brain works differently in ADHD. This can lead to delaying engagement with those tasks until an absolute deadline approaches (that hyperbolic behaviour again).

This happens for different reasons. One is that our brain's reward centre will often push us towards other palatable alternatives (such as doom scrolling on a phone), but we might also choose so-called aversive alternatives, such as cleaning the house. This is the basis of James' joke about aversive distractions from Chapter 8 that if you want your house cleaned, just ask somebody with ADHD to do their actual job (he is only partly joking with this advice!).

What this means is that our engagement with the task can only be improved by finding ways to stop these two procrastination forms. For active procrastination, we can split a task into shorter, meaningful and achievable milestones. This means that there are several 'absolute deadlines' spread out a bit, like writing single book chapters instead of writing a whole book. For passive procrastination, the key is to increase the emotional reward for doing the task you want to achieve (such as making someone you care about happy), while removing the opportunity for those easy, more palatable options (such as deleting certain apps on your phone or having a set time every day when you allow yourself to doom scroll).

A contributing factor to both active and passive procrastination is distractibility. ADHD is obviously an issue with attention (it is in the name) and includes a strong neurological tendency to be easily distracted. Although distractibility is intrinsically linked to reward, it can be viewed as a separate influencing factor. When trying to engage with any task, distraction (and crucially an environment in which we can be distracted) can lead to serious procrastination.

We imagine this isn't surprising if you have ADHD. This could be anything from having multiple tabs open on an internet browser to having a mobile phone close to hand. It can even be a challenge having a glass window in front of you, through which you can see pretty much anything at all. This often provides stronger immediate feelings of reward than the thought of completing the task we are trying to engage with.

When we coach people with ADHD who are struggling with procrastination, one of the first questions we ask is, 'What can you see around you at your workstation?' If the answer includes items such as general clutter, multiple screens and devices, and even that window, it is easy to understand why they are procrastinating – there are so many available alternatives to doing the task right in front of their nose. Combine distractibility with poor working memory, and one can very quickly forget that there was something that needed to be done in the first place. Optimising your workspace can be a sensible first step in trying to block distractions and activities that compete for your attention.

Finally, an interesting (sort of) theory of procrastination is called the temporal motivation theory. We know that ADHD adults often have a different pacing style for tasks, which means we seek out immediate reward over delayed reward, we have an intention-action gap (if you remember, this means that people with ADHD can struggle to convert what we intend to do into an action) and we are often less likely to be able to resist tempting distractions and random thoughts. This temporal motivation theory suggests that time blindness is central to this problem. Because we struggle to see something (such as a project due) even relatively soon as in any way relevant to us right now, it can be difficult for us to visualise a deadline in the distant future, so non-imminent tasks can fade into the background of importance completely. We nearly didn't include that explanation in case we didn't get it exactly correct, which introduces us the challenge of...

Perfectionism

Perfectionism is somewhere between 'a form of anxiety' and 'a personality trait'. A balanced amount of perfectionism can be a positive trait, motivating people to achieve their goals and produce high-quality work. More often, however, this is a tendency to set extremely (often unrealistically) high standards for oneself, to strive for absolute flawlessness, having a crippling fear of perceived failure or having very self-critical tendencies.

This kind of perfectionism can have negative consequences (especially when driven by a fear of failure), leading to procrastination, anxiety and depression. Holding unrealistic performance standards can delay the completion of a task until those standards are met, sometimes leading to projects remaining unfinished forever. This means that perfectionism can be a core reason for procrastination and has been reported (maybe surprisingly) as the most common 'cognitive distortion' (irrational thought process) seen in people with ADHD.[100] It may seem counter-intuitive, but research has also shown that impulsivity and perfectionism co-occur in ADHD. We don't know why.

Perfectionism comes in two main types: front-end perfectionism (having rigid standards or preconditions that must be met to engage in a task in the first place) and back-end perfectionism (which sounds rude, but means having extremely high and rigid standards for quality and details). Anecdotally, front-end perfectionism is more common in ADHD (possibly due to RSD), but ultimately both forms of perfectionism can be viewed as a protective mechanism for dealing with potential future criticism.

Productivity

The challenges of prioritisation, procrastination and perfectionism that we have discussed in this chapter combine with all those other elements of ADHD and very often lead to reduced productivity in the workplace (and everywhere else – except for that random hobby that you have had for a few weeks now).

It is important to reiterate that this doesn't mean having ADHD always leads to an unproductive worker. With the right support in place, we are told that people with ADHD can be incredibly productive (not personally, so far, but we live in hope). Without that support, however, the impact of those issues with prioritisation, procrastination and perfectionism can be serious and significant barriers to success and productivity. One study even quantified this as a 4–5 per cent reduction in workplace performance for those with unsupported ADHD.[101]

One common definition of productivity is: 'The ability of an individual to complete tasks or accomplish goals efficiently and effectively. It is a measure of how much output an individual can produce with a given amount of input.' For many people with ADHD, their output might actually be the same (or greater) than their colleagues' output, but due to a lack of boundaries, impostor syndrome and the factors mentioned above, the input often has to be higher to achieve this level. This means that many people with ADHD have to work harder to achieve the same 'success', and a study by the World Health Organization reported that untreated ADHD adults lose an average of 22 days of productivity per year.[102]

ADHD & THE 4 P's

When we refer to 'productivity', we are mostly describing outputs that you individually want to do and value. We know all too well that ADHD people are stigmatised more because of how society fetishes hyper-productivity and the amount of time people spend at work. Human value should not be measured in output units, and productivity should include how you made people feel. Having said that, if adults with ADHD were more supported, there would be fewer issues with productivity. It is frustrating that a lack of support is one of the key reasons why we face reduced employment, as well as increased risk of burnout and workplace stress. According to one (admittedly small) study, we are 75 per cent more likely to face long-term sickness absence and 25 per cent of people on long-term sickness absence leave may have ADHD.[103] As well as affecting the individual employee, this means there are unnecessary, associated costs to employers and the economy that a relatively cheap level of diagnosis and support could mitigate. A 2012 report estimated costs of adult ADHD to the US economy alone of $38 billion to $72 billion per year.[104]

If adults with ADHD were appropriately diagnosed, treated, managed and supported in the workplace, they would have the same chance of being able to perform their job to the same degree as anyone else, without the increased risk of burnout. People with ADHD often take the blame for workplace issues, when it is employers who should be asking themselves, 'Would we support employees who had a visible disability?' We are sure that most employers would say yes to this, so why not support ADHD appropriately?

SUMMARY

If you want to be productive and get something done, you have to know why you are doing it and what to do first. You also need to have a measure of success clear in your head. Perfect is the enemy of good, so you need to know what constitutes a good-enough job. Even if you know what to do first, you need to be able to start that task and then persevere until that job is finished. People with ADHD often face problems with all of this.

Problems with prioritisation, perfectionism and procrastination arise because of the differences in the brain's executive functions. We know that all of those executive elements of our brain that direct our ability to manage tasks, focus attention and control our impulses can lead to decreased productivity. But with the right strategies and support, adults with ADHD can overcome those productivity barriers and start to write goals in line with their different way of doing things.

Putting all of those strategies into practice is difficult enough with ADHD on its own. Despite that challenge, four out of every five adults with ADHD are living with at least one other health condition, and this exacerbates and complicates how we move forward and which support would be helpful. We call this ADHD plus. In the next and penultimate chapter, we want to explain the main conditions that commonly coexist with ADHD, how that can make things even more complicated and hopefully, give you some ideas on how to move forward as an individual.

CHAPTER 15

ADHD+: comorbidities

If you are an adult with ADHD reading this and you ONLY have ADHD, you are in the significant minority. As many as 80 per cent of us have one or more extra coexisting conditions (also called comorbidities).[105] The term we use for this in our community is ADHD Plus or ADHD+. CHADD, the leading American non-profit organisation for people affected by ADHD, has written a useful summary of the main mental health conditions and learning differences faced by people with ADHD.[106]

There are many coexisting conditions in the ADHD+™ stable, such as mood disorder, anxiety and other neurodivergences such as autism (or autistic traits), tics and learning differences. There are also lots of other conditions or disorders we are born with or that develop later in life.[107] Some of these coexist by chance (as they might for anybody else), but others are statistically more likely to occur if you have ADHD. We don't always know why.

Sometimes, the existence of a second condition is a coincidence, but in other cases the second condition could be linked to having ADHD. This link could be due to your brain biology, or it could have arisen directly because of living with ADHD and the effect of growing up with ADHD in society. It may even be all of those factors combined in some people or due to a shared but unrelated factor in others (brilliantly called a confounding variable). It is quite complicated and everyone is different.

It might interest you to know that many people use the term 'coexisting condition' because the term 'comorbidity' appears a bit dark and linked to death, possibly because of the word mortality. In actual fact, the word 'comorbid' comes from the Latin for 'together' and 'illness' not 'death' at all (which is 'mort' in Latin). What we do know is that there appears to be evidence for both physical AND mental comorbid (or coexisting) conditions associated more strongly with ADHD. Let's start with the relatively less well studied and probably smaller group of physical conditions.

Physical coexisting conditions linked to ADHD

People with ADHD seem to be more likely to have physical conditions than the general population.[108] This is fascinating, but there isn't a lot known about why this might be. We don't fully know if these are statistical links due to coincidental factors (such as ADHD being linked to a lower (average) wage and therefore worse healthcare), or if there are physical conditions that have real, biological connections to ADHD. In most cases, there seems to be a shared genetic factor, but in others (such as an increased risk of nervous system disorders), these conditions probably arise

ADHD+: COMORBIDITIES

due to a common environment more than the same biology. Some of the more frequently reported physical challenges connected to ADHD are sleep disorders, epilepsy and dementia, as well as muscular and metabolic problems and asthma (and other breathing issues).

Some of the statistical links to ADHD are small differences (such as a 2 per cent chance of having a pre-existing heart disorder for children with ADHD, compared with 1.2 per cent more widely).[109] That last research actually looked at 'children who were treated with methylphenidate' rather than children with ADHD, but of course that experiment could then be reported as an effect of taking Ritalin rather than a link to having ADHD (a great example of how poor science reporting can lead to unhelpful scaremongering).

Some physical disorders might have the same biological basis as the developmental changes in the ADHD brain. One possible example of this would be restless leg syndrome (RLS), although it could also be true that because RLS is often triggered or exacerbated by sleep disorders (which are far more common in people with ADHD), it is a confounding variable rather than a shared biology.[110] What is more compelling is the link between ADHD and hypermobility (extremely flexible joints and limbs).

Hypermobility and ADHD

We get asked a lot about a possible link between ADHD and extreme joint flexibility, presumably because many people have noticed the link in their own family. This is sometimes called hypermobility and includes one particularly nasty hypermobile condition called Ehlers–Danlos syndrome (EDS). We have also noticed that we are meeting an increasing number of   people who are both hypermobile and who have ADHD; it seems a lot more than we would expect by chance. There may even be a causal link between the likely causes of hypermobile joints and the changes to our brain structure.[111] As both involve physical connections requiring connective tissue, this could be the genetic reason in some ADHD people (this isn't proven – rather our semi-educated guess). What we know is that several studies show large and significant differences in the numbers of ADHD people (compared to the general population) having hypermobility in general[112] and in Ehlers–Danlos syndrome specifically.[113]

Mental health conditions linked to ADHD

Usually, when we talk about conditions that coexist with ADHD (that 80 per cent figure), we are mostly referring to other mental health conditions (or differences, of course, if you prefer). Some of these other conditions may have arisen directly BECAUSE of living with ADHD, whereas others might be part of your individual profile for the same biological reason that you developed ADHD (your genetic, neurodevelopmental make-up). Others still may be entirely coincidental, because we are as likely as any member of the general population to get a medical condition (ADHD sadly doesn't stop you from getting other medical conditions).

In some cases, however, it isn't a coincidence, and we are more likely to face other illnesses and conditions. It is also important to say that you will probably never know which

ADHD+: COMORBIDITIES

of the above reasons is your individual one for having an increased burden. For example, we could have an anxiety disorder separate from ADHD or directly because of living with ADHD.

There is no limit to the possible mental health conditions that can coexist with ADHD but Tourette's is the most common one by quite some distance. It has been estimated that more than 60 per cent of children with Tourette's will develop ADHD.[114] Sleep problems are also common among people with ADHD, with a number of (admittedly wide-ranging) estimates from 25–65 per cent of people with ADHD reporting sleep disturbance.[115] These are challenging because (you may well know from personal experience) insomnia and other sleep disorders can exacerbate ADHD symptoms and severely impact overall mental health. Another frequent occurrence is the presence of autistic traits or autism together with ADHD (sometimes described as AuDHD). There is a large subgroup of people with AuDHD, and while some of the symptoms overlap, others (such as craving routine and being easily bored) can clash, causing some particularly difficult challenges for living peacefully.

Anxiety and depressive disorders, such as generalised anxiety disorder (GAD), social phobia and panic disorder, often coexist with ADHD, and this can make things more challenging. People with ADHD may experience heightened levels of anxiety due to difficulties with organisation, time management and task completion. Or it may be because of how ADHD makes us feel being weak in these areas when society values them so highly. We find the anxiety form of social phobia particularly interesting, as it isn't just the fear of being in a crowd. It is an intense, persistent fear of being (or feeling) watched and judged by others, which may well tie in with rejection sensitivity (see Chapter 11 for a reminder of that horrible nightmare).

Depression is another mood disorder that can often occur alongside ADHD, particularly in adults. In fact, many adults with ADHD have dysthymia, which is a milder but more long-lasting form of depression. The challenges and frustrations associated with managing ADHD symptoms can contribute to feelings of sadness and hopelessness. With both anxiety and depression (and many others), there is a chicken and egg problem to think about. It is notoriously difficult to know if the anxiety is because of the ADHD, if it is entirely unrelated (thanks universe) or, more worryingly, if the effect of having anxiety (for example) and ADHD together is worse than these conditions would be individually. The chicken PLUS egg scenario has an unpleasant synergy that lets the analogy down a bit.

Despite addiction sometimes relating to self-medication with drugs or alcohol as a coping mechanism for managing ADHD-related symptoms, psychologists tend to include substance use disorders (SUDs) as a coexisting condition. People with ADHD are at a higher risk of developing substance use disorders, especially in adolescence and adulthood. Other addictions (or repetitive behaviours such as gambling, sexual addiction or impulse spending) may also reflect the reward centre of ADHD being affected.

People with ADHD often report a history of misdiagnoses. This is particularly complicated because a number of coexisting conditions are more likely to be seen with ADHD but also with some overlapping symptoms. One example would be the emotional dysregulation (or mood swings) of bipolar disorder (BD), often seeing overlap with some of the impulsive and hyperactive behaviours of people with ADHD. Another example includes the group of specific learning disabilities (SPLD), such as dyslexia or dyscalculia. Not only do these share some symptoms (such as not being able to concentrate on reading), but you might even see ADHD included as an SPLD in general, even in some places where they should know better.

ADHD isn't a specific learning difficulty. While one person's individual ADHD *could* be a specific learning difference, it isn't at all accurate to say that of all ADHD. If you are struggling to explain why to someone, you can just ask them the very simple question, 'What is the specific thing that all adults with ADHD can't learn?' There isn't an answer to that question so therefore it isn't an SPLD.

A few so-called personality disorders are also more likely to coexist with ADHD. We don't love the term 'personality disorder' and think it creates unhelpful stigmas, but at the moment these are the names we are expected to use from a medical perspective. These disorders are a step beyond the typical ADHD behaviours, such as pathological demand avoidance (PDA, but also known as extreme demand avoidance or EDA) or a general response to fears of rejection – these are something far more aggressive or hostile. Some of them, such as oppositional defiant disorder (ODD) or conduct disorder (CD) are labels often given to children (and teenagers) to reflect quite extreme patterns of defiant, antisocial, disobedient and/or hostile behaviour toward authority figures. These are rare but we have noticed that they often lead to an additional ADHD diagnosis and might reflect why people tend to think of ADHD as 'naughty children'. In adults, these tend to develop into serious conditions sometimes (possibly unhelpfully) referred to as borderline personality disorder or narcissistic personality disorder.

Societal conditions

Untreated and unmanaged, ADHD can lead to more socio-economic difficulties than the average population faces. Financial problems and other societal challenges, such as relationship issues, criminality and poverty, can have health impacts of their own.

Increased impact

Even for those conditions that aren't statistically more likely, being comorbid with ADHD can have a bigger effect on someone with ADHD than it does on someone without, leading to (and we quote) 'severe impairment of everyday life with considerable functional and psychosocial problems'.[116] That last quote is particularly notable as James knew at some point that Alex would have to embarrassingly shoehorn a reference to a paper from 2010 that he co-authored, pointing out that we need to look at the impact of these coexisting conditions on the symptom progression of people with ADHD.[117]

SUMMARY

Although most people with ADHD have a coexisting condition, one in five of us don't. For the rest of us, the exact combination of conditions can vary widely from person to person. This means that accurate diagnosis and comprehensive assessment are essential for developing a tailored treatment plan that addresses ADHD within your personal profile and life.

Treatment options may include therapy, medication, lifestyle modifications and support from mental health professionals. There is no doubt that the challenge of living with coexisting conditions (ADHD+) adds increased stress and complexity to a community already finding the easy things more difficult and facing stigma. While this is clearly yet another challenge to deal with, the important thing is to include ADHD+ in every conversation from school to work. It isn't really necessary (or even possible) to split behaviours into an ADHD part and a different part (as with personality in general). Instead, treat ADHD+ as another element with individual support needs and societal pressures.

It is hard to balance the obvious need for support for our ADHD, whether on its own or ADHD+ and the pragmatic reality that we are very much in the minority, facing challenges of living and thriving in a neurotypical world. In the last chapter, we will look at navigating that environment and hopefully give you some ideas and tips on how to survive in a world that feels designed for people who seem to be very different to us.

CHAPTER 16

How to navigate a neurotypical world

We may have already said in this book, but as a reminder we don't actually like using the word 'neurotypical' to describe individual people. This is because nobody is exactly 'typical', it is a hypothetical average and it seems to be used a bit unkindly to describe (often fictitiously) common behaviours of people without ADHD. Lots of our family and friends don't have ADHD and they are all different.

Having said that, the majority of people in the world aren't neurodivergent, meaning they are more likely to think and behave 'within typical parameters'. Societal norms and expectations have been developed to encompass this and we refer to that as neurotypical, rather than individual people. What is considered 'normal', 'appropriate' and 'desirable' is very often based around those typical parameters and traits, which excludes those who don't fit into these constraints. People often mistakenly refer to that as 'normal'.

Because of the persistent and damaging stigmas associated with ADHD, most people spend a big portion of their lives before diagnosis masking their symptoms (and very often after diagnosis, to be honest). Masking (as we see it) is the process of unhealthily concealing or suppressing symptoms and traits to 'blend in' with social or professional environments. There is a blurred line between more healthy coping strategies to protect ourselves (such as choosing who to discuss our diagnosis with) and the stressful suppression of ourselves seen in masking, but we will try and point that out when it arises.

Often, masking is driven by exposure to previous criticism, fear of stigma or being judged, or not wanting to feel or appear to be 'different'. Although it is sometimes seen as a positive (usually from the outside), masking very often leads to significant psychological stress, a negative self-image and an exacerbation of symptoms. While masking isn't unique to ADHD (it is more well-known in the autistic community), its impact on the ADHD community is profound. Masking can lead to increased stress, anxiety and even depression because the effort needed to hide our true selves or to meet perceived societal standards is both exhausting and inauthentic. Importantly, masking can and often does delay the diagnosis and treatment of ADHD, as people may not present as 'typical' ADHD cases due to how well they mask their symptoms.

Examples of masking include over-preparing for social interactions to avoid appearing forgetful or disorganised, even to the point of compulsively rehearsing potential conversations and trips, suppressing our natural tendencies towards external hyperactivity (often annoyingly referred to as fidgeting) or impulsiveness in settings where such behaviours are deemed inappropriate. Both of us used to sit in meetings where it wasn't seen as appropriate to move around. Alex would bite the inside of his mouth until it bled to avoid standing or interrupting (why is it seen as such a bad thing to have to walk around occasionally?). We would also sit on our hands, but we never questioned WHY this was wrong. We just saw how everyone else behaved and internalised that as the correct way to act.

Remember we are 'normal'; we are just not typical. In the same way that very tall people are not a typical height but are still, of course, normal people. Despite that, the mimicking of others' behaviours, routines or work habits in an attempt to appear more 'normal' or to fit in better is common, and trying to react how we might be 'expected to' (even though it often isn't how we want to react) is tiring and usually unnecessary.

Masking isn't free. This isn't just a case of wanting to do or say whatever we want without having to obey any rules. Of course, we all need a range of useful tools for navigating social and professional situations, and these are healthy social strategies. However, feeling the need to forcefully suppress many of our needs and behaviours, comes at a cost, especially when it becomes a consistent strategy for 'fitting in'. Constantly monitoring and adjusting our behaviour to appear 'typical' can be incredibly stressful and can counterproductively exacerbate ADHD symptoms.

Over time, masking often leads to questioning our identity. Many people don't realise or accept they have ADHD because they mask so well. They don't even consider what their symptoms (or preferences) would be like 'unmasked'. The internal strain of masking can lead to feelings of isolation, and the effort required to constantly mask symptoms can be emotionally draining, contributing to the risk of burnout and other mental illnesses.

Adults with ADHD are often 'square pegs'. We don't quite fit into the round holes that society expects of us, so we force ourselves to act the way we think 'other people' act in order to squeeze ourselves into those round holes. What does this tell us? That society needs to start making square holes because, and we can't stress this enough, *we deserve to be ourselves*. And if society won't make square holes, we will make them ourselves.

Emotional acceptance

On our podcast, The ADHD Adults,[118] we have a running joke of saying 'Emotional acceptance blah blah blah' because we say it so often that it has become repetitive. The reason we say it so often is because this is one of the most powerful tools in learning to defang the impact that ADHD can have on a day-to-day basis. And the reason why we don't just call it acceptance is because there are different ways in which we can accept things. To cognitively accept that we have ADHD is relatively easy. Emotionally accepting ADHD is often more challenging.

Emotional acceptance involves recognising and accepting that basic fact that we don't choose to be forgetful or distractible, that there is a reason we may make mistakes or impulsively buy something and that it isn't a weakness of character or a question of willpower. Acceptance enables people to approach their condition with more compassion and understanding, possibly leading to better self-care and a more positive outlook on life. Emotional acceptance of ADHD, which can take years even after diagnosis, enables us to reduce the self-chastisement that often feeds low self-esteem and impostor syndrome. This self-chastisement amplifies the impact that ADHD symptoms and traits can have on our mental health, relationships and functioning.

Adults with ADHD often experience this negative self-talk due to repeated 'failures' or difficulties in completing daily tasks. As ADHD coaches, one statement we hear (and have thought) very often is, 'I don't feel like a proper adult.' Emotional acceptance helps in recognising these negative patterns and can help to foster a more compassionate self-view, reducing the impact of our internal negative bias. Fundamentally understanding that the difficulties we face are a part of a disorder (or condition, whichever you identify as having), rather than a personal failure, can dial down that negative self-talk.

Emotional acceptance can also help to build resilience. Resilience is an odd concept in ADHD. Social media is full of posts stating that adults with ADHD are resilient, when in fact resilience – the ability to bounce back quickly from adversity – is often very difficult with ADHD. Emotional acceptance can help to reduce stress and anxiety, making it easier to navigate difficulties with daily tasks and social interactions.

Two approaches that anecdotally can help include trying to find the humour in everyday ADHDing, and in the early stage of your ADHD 'journey' using something as a totem (such as a wristband). This is a physical object that you can touch as a reminder to help you mentally step back and accept that you don't always have to carry the responsibility for how your brain works.

These elements are true for almost everyone with ADHD in every aspect of our lives. There are also some specific things you can try for work and home. Some of them require communicating your needs with others. We always want to be as authentic as possible, but we also have to survive in a very neurotypical world, meaning the choice of how open to be with colleagues, teachers and friends depends from person to person. Deciding what to share and what to keep private can depend on the support around us.

Thriving with ADHD in professional and social settings

A lot of change is happening right now as employers, schools and families are learning more about the reality of ADHD. We know that some of this isn't great and it could be a lot quicker and more evidence-led, but as people who have been living with this for decades, we do see a positive development. Unfortunately, we (as an ADHD community) seem to be the ones tasked with understanding, navigating and sometimes explaining how people with ADHD can be supported. We can moan about that (and we do – a lot), but it is also helpful to talk about those support options here.

Professional environment

We strongly believe that, where possible, 'coming out' as someone with ADHD benefits most people in the workplace, not least in that it usually provides legal protection from discrimination. The thing is, the feeling of 'safety' and 'power' needed to declare our ADHD in the first place can be disappointingly rare. We would never be able to more generally advise people to disclose their ADHD because legal protections aren't as safe as they should be.

Frustratingly, one of the reasons why disclosure can be good is that it makes it easier to ask for reasonable changes (or accommodations) to remove some of those structural barriers. This could even be an informal conversation with HR or an occupational health professional. There is no specific list of accommodations, as we are all different, but we have tried to come up with a few common requests here.

IDEAS FOR ADHD ACCOMMODATIONS

1. Many workplaces are required to provide reasonable accommodations for employees with disabilities, including ADHD. This might include flexible scheduling, a quiet workspace or the ability to use headphones to listen to music while working. Some people with ADHD are so distracted by others that 'hot-desking', where we never have a fixed office space, is absolutely unworkable. However, for some of us (such as Alex) who really struggle with quiet offices, hot-desking works quite well.

2. Digital tools and apps designed for task management can be particularly helpful. Features such as reminders, timers and calendars can help you stay on track with deadlines and meetings. Try different ones and see if they work for you.

3. Large projects can be overwhelming. Breaking them down into more manageable tasks can help maintain focus and momentum. This is a fundamental of ADHD success (S.M.A.R.T goals might be a place to start; see below).

4. Agreeing to a validation conversation can also be really helpful. Many employers and managers don't understand the value of a simple 'thumbs-up' to let us know we are valued. We are not suggesting a three-hour weekly meeting and hugs – it could be just a small, regular reminder that we are not completely useless or failing. This can be a huge benefit to the vast numbers of adults with ADHD who are struggling with rejection sensitivity and the need for clear external validation.

Setting S.M.A.R.T goals

We've talked a few times about breaking tasks down. It is very useful to make a task clearly 'winnable' by knowing exactly what tiny thing you have to do first (that IS the task, the next step is a second task). You also have to be clear how to do it, and know whether it is actually realistic. There are no rules for this but we quite like the S.M.A.R.T goal model where you make each task for the S.M.A.R.T acronym:

- **Specific**: Know what a win looks like. Make this as small a task as possible.

- **Measurable**: Will you know you have won? (Tidying up is never measurable, emptying a dishwasher is.)

- **Achievable**: Are you able to do this task?

- **Realistic**: Even if you are able, is it realistic for you here and now?

- **Time-bound**: Do you have time? Do you know how long it will take? Have you assigned time to this?

Social settings

Sometimes, asking for adjustments at work can be simpler than in social and family settings. We can blame the need for 'productivity' or 'profit'. The effect on adults with ADHD socially is very complex and emotionally charged (whether we have other coexisting social challenges or not). As always, communication and control seem to be the most useful elements to live more peacefully.

Firstly, remember you have control: engage in social activities that align with your interests and strengths. Settings in which you feel comfortable and engaged can reduce social anxiety and make interactions more enjoyable. If you need to put a time limit on a gathering, that is OK. If you need a relaxing, fun activity (such as watching a film) to also be a task to tick off a list, that is OK. It isn't shameful to want to play the guitar or chat to a friend AND think that it is a task that needs to be done. That is ADHD.

Most importantly, communicate your needs and plans, especially when these will affect other people: don't hesitate to let friends know which environments or situations are challenging for you. A true friend will understand and may even help you navigate social settings more comfortably. Explaining in advance that you might leave a party early (especially if you struggle with substance use) or might not be comfortable watching an entire film in one sitting can reduce that shame and stop people from thinking it is their company (or choice of film) causing you discomfort.

Managing daily life

The key to staying in control with ADHD is routine and structure, which you have both chosen and have control over, and which might not be logical from the outside. This might adapt as you learn more and develop in your ADHD life. The lifelong challenge is trying to find a routine (as James puts it) 'in the sweet spot between rigidity and flexibility'. Trying and failing IS a success because you learn about yourself.

Establishing a consistent routine can be incredibly difficult, but it can support us with time management and reduce the chances of forgetting important tasks or appointments. Yet again, trying and failing at new structures and routines is the key to success. We learn what doesn't work, or what only works in certain situations. Accepting this enables us to move on, trying new ideas until we have a massive arsenal of personal structures and routines that sometimes work for us. Embrace failure and try something else.

When it comes to health and wellness, most of us know that regular exercise, adequate sleep and a nutritious diet can significantly impact our ability to manage ADHD symptoms. Physical activity, in particular, has been shown to reduce symptoms of ADHD. But how do we know what to do and keep it going?

As with most ADHD elements, form follows function. If you have to force yourself to do a certain sport, it might not be the one for you. Some people hate running but will happily play tennis, go dancing or join a gym. Others can only do online fitness, and some actually like running. There is no value in self-criticism for what your brain prefers. As with the routines and structures above, try different things and see what feels the easiest. There are structural barriers in society that restrict access to health and well-being, but the one you have more control of is choosing activities that feel positive for you as an individual. Alex likes trail running with obstacles and mud, for example (that should be a separate diagnosis!).

Seeking support

Whether you think ADHD is just a difference to be celebrated, a problem with modern society or a neurological disability, every single one of us can be more successful and internally peaceful with a bit more support. The nature of that support depends on the person but please give yourself time to really think about what could be useful.

There is a general feeling in society that we 'should' be able to just get on with things without professional help or medication. But this 'keep calm and carry on' approach simply isn't working. If it was, the burdens of ADHD we have discussed a lot in this book wouldn't be there, and they certainly wouldn't decrease with treatment. But they do.

Seek professional help too. A therapist who specialises in ADHD can provide valuable strategies tailored to your specific challenges and needs. The relationship between the therapist and the client (or patient) is one of the most important elements in positive change. Chat with them about their perspective on ADHD and share how you feel about it. If, like us, you want a positive lens but see ADHD as a disorder, avoid a therapist who focuses on superpowers. If you feel your ADHD is a fantastic, creative gift, work with someone who feels the same way.

We are ADHD coaches, which is in no way medical or a therapy. BUT there is growing evidence that people feel supported by ADHD coaching and that ADHD coaches can help with some of the key daily challenges such as procrastination, productivity and goal setting. Again, the right coach for you personally is the most important part of the conversation.

Medication may also be an option worth exploring with a healthcare provider. ADHD medication can be effective for a few key elements of ADHD in most of us, but this is not a cure and the medicines can cause a few side effects (too many to list, but dry mouth and loss of appetite can be common).

Regardless of your position and access to ADHD meds, the talking treatment and social support are still fundamental needs. If you can't access individual support, there are lots of support groups both online and within our communities. Connecting with others who have ADHD can provide a sense of community, understanding and shared experiences. Support groups can be a great resource for tips and strategies that have worked for others.

Educate others

Where appropriate, educating friends, family and colleagues about ADHD can help them understand your experiences and behaviours. This can foster a supportive environment and reduce misunderstandings. Maybe ... erm ... buy them a book on the subject. Shameless plug!

What next?

So here we are. You have either got this far or skipped straight to the last paragraphs. We are very lucky that we get to hear from thousands of people living with their ADHD and although there are common themes, every story is different and reassuringly relatable. We know that understanding more about ADHD only opens up a lot more questions. But we also know that being empowered and sharing can help us live with our ADHD more healthily. It can help us with the crucial emotional acceptance. And it can help us talk more about our challenges and accept the support that is available.

As you navigate the neurotypical world, including managing your ADHD traits of inattention or hyperactivity/impulsivity on a day-to-day basis, reducing harmful masking and learning coping strategies to help with executive function, or embracing new and exciting ways to build closer relationships, it is important to keep in mind that *you are the expert in your ADHD*. You are the only person who truly understands your specific circumstances and how ADHD affects you as an individual.

As you move through life with the challenges of ADHD, you will flex some interesting muscles and develop some highly useful coping strategies. These skills are often honed because other people didn't have to learn them. That is the real superpower, so think about what you are good at and what is healthy for you. Remember, you have strengths and qualities that make you *more* than your ADHD. You are the cake, not the ingredients. You are unique, but you are not alone. We are legion, and our voices are starting to be heard.

References

1. Hommel B, Chapman CS, Cisek P et al, 'No one knows what attention is', *Atten Percept Psychophys*, vol. 81, pages 2288–2303, 2019. doi: 10.3758/s13414-019-01846-w
2. *Diagnostic and Statistical Manual of Mental Disorders* (5th ed.), American Psychiatric Association, 2013. https://doi.org/10.1176/appi.books.9780890425596
3. Still, GF, 'The Goulstonian lectures on some abnormal psychical conditions in children', *The Lancet*, vol. 159, pages 1008–1013, London, 1902. https://doi.org/10.1016/S0140-6736(01)74984-7
4. 'How many people in the UK have diabetes?' Diabetes UK, accessed September 2024. https://www.diabetes.org.uk/about-us/about-the-charity/our-strategy/statistics
5. Faraone SV et al, 'The World Federation of ADHD International Consensus Statement: 208 Evidence-based conclusions about the disorder', *Neuroscience & Biobehavioral Reviews*, vol. 128, pages 789–818, 2021. https://doi.org/10.1016/j.neubiorev.2021.01.022.
6. Popit S, Serod K, Locatelli I, Stuhec M, 'Prevalence of attention-deficit hyperactivity disorder (ADHD): systematic review and meta-analysis', *Eur Psychiatry.* 2024 Oct 9;67(1):e68. doi: 10.1192/j.eurpsy.2024.1786. PMID: 39381949
7. Dale D et al, 'The economic burden of adult attention deficit hyperactivity disorder: A sibling comparison cost analysis', *European Psychiatry: the Journal of the European Psychiatric Association,* vol. 61, pages 41–48, 2019. doi: 10.1016/j.eurpsy.2019.06.011
8. Gershman SJ and Ullman TD, 'Causal implicatures from correlational statements', *PLoS One*, vol. 18(5), e0286067, 2019. doi: 10.1371/journal.pone.0286067
9. Digital G, 'Autism increase mystery solved? No, it's not vaccines, GMOs, glyphosate—or organic foods', *Genetic Literacy Project*, 2023. https://geneticliteracyproject.org/2023/11/13/autism-increase-mystery-solved-no-its-not-vaccines-gmos-glyphosate-or-organic-foods
10. Støy J, De Franco E, Ye H et al, 'In celebration of a century with insulin – Update of insulin gene mutations in diabetes', *Mol Metab*, vol. 52, page 101280, 2021. doi: 10.1016/j.molmet.2021.101280
11. Grimm O, Kranz TM and Reif A, 'Genetics of ADHD: What should the

clinician know?', *Current Psychiatry Reports*, vol. *22*(4), page 18, 2020. https://doi.org/10.1007/s11920-020-1141-x

12. Stevens SE, Kumsta R, Kreppner JM et al, 'Dopamine transporter gene polymorphism moderates the effects of severe deprivation on ADHD symptoms: developmental continuities in gene-environment interplay', *Am J Med Genet B Neuropsychiatr Genet*, vol. 150B (6), pages 753–61, 2009. doi: 10.1002/ajmg.b.31010

13. Severe childhood deprivation has longstanding impacts on brain size in adulthood,' King's College London, 2020. https://www.kcl.ac.uk/news/severe-childhood-deprivation-has-longstanding-impacts-on-brain-size-in-adulthood

14. 'Position Statement on therapies focused on memories of childhood physical and sexual abuse', American Psychiatric Association, Board of Trustees, Assembly & APA Operations Manual, 2000. https://www.psychiatry.org/getattachment/930fb215-2147-40e9-9d44-f06d84fc-64de/Position-2013-Memories-Child-Abuse.pdf

15. Herculano-Houzel S, 'The remarkable, yet not extraordinary, human brain as a scaled-up primate brain and its associated cost', *Proceedings of the National Academy of Sciences*, vol. 109 (supplement_1), pages 10661–10668, 2012. doi:10.1073/pnas.1201895109.

16. Lange KW, Reichl S, Lange KM et al, 'The history of attention deficit hyperactivity disorder', *Atten Defic Hyperact Disord*, vol. 2(4), pages 241–55, 2010. doi: 10.1007/s12402-010-0045-8.

17. Lawson D, 'I'm sorry, but all this ADHD doesn't add up', *The Sunday Times*, 5 February 2023. https://www.thetimes.co.uk/article/all-this-a-dhd-doesnt-add-up-comment-vqvl9kqvn.

18. Vening J, 'I may not be a doctor ... but I'm almost certain you have ADHD', *The Guardian*, 3 November 2022. https://www.theguardian.com/commentisfree/2022/nov/04/i-may-not-be-a-doctor-but-i-am-almost-certain-you-have-adhd.

19. Coren G, 'I'm calm and focused for this ADHD test...', *The Times*, 10 February 2023. https://www.thetimes.co.uk/article/im-calm-and-focused-for-this-adhd-test-58v63w8hq.

20. Faraone SV, Banaschewski T, Coghill D et al, 'The World Federation of ADHD International Consensus Statement: 208 Evidence-based conclusions about the disorder', *Neuroscience & Biobehavioral Reviews*, vol. 128, pages 789–818, 2021. https://doi.org/10.1016/j.neubiorev.2021.01.022.

21. Taylor E, 'Antecedents of ADHD: a historical account of diagnostic concepts', *Adhd Attention Deficit and Hyperactivity Disorders*, vol. 3(2), pages 69–75, (2011). https://doi.org/10.1007/s12402-010-0051-x.

22. Arnold LE, Hodgkins P and Kewley G, 'Long-term outcomes of ADHD: academic achievement and performance', *Journal of Attention Disorders*, vol. 24(1), pages 73–85, 2015. https://doi.org/10.1177/1087054714566076.

23. Conner A and Brown J, 'Adult ADHD and higher education: improving the

REFERENCES

student experience', *Times Higher Education*, 31 January 2022. https://www.timeshighereducation.com/campus/adult-adhd-and-higher-education-improving-student-experience

24. Kooij JJS, Bejerot S, Blackwell A et al, 'European consensus statement on diagnosis and treatment of adult ADHD: The European Network Adult ADHD', *BMC Psychiatry*, vol. 10(1), article 67, 2010. https://doi.org/10.1186/1471-244x-10-67.

25. Palladino VS, McNeill R, Reif A and Kittel-Schneider S, 'Genetic risk factors and gene–environment interactions in adult and childhood attention-deficit/hyperactivity disorder', *Psychiatric Genetics*, vol. 29(3), pages 63–78, 2019). https://doi.org/10.1097/ypg.0000000000000220.

26. Shi Y, Hunter Guevara, LR, Dykhoff HJ et al, 'Racial Disparities in Diagnosis of Attention-Deficit/Hyperactivity Disorder in a US National Birth Cohort', *JAMA Network Open*, vol. 4(3), page e210321, 2021. https://doi.org/10.1001/jamanetworkopen.2021.0321.

27. Abé C, Rahman Q, Långström N et al, 'Cortical brain structure and sexual orientation in adult females with bipolar disorder or attention deficit hyperactivity disorder', *Brain and Behavior*, vol. 8(7), page e00998, 2018. https://doi.org/10.1002/brb3.998

28. Strang J, Kenworthy L, Dominska A et al, 'Increased gender variance in autism spectrum disorders and attention deficit hyperactivity disorder', *Archives of Sexual Behavior*, vol. 43(8), pages 1525–1533, 2014. https://doi.org/10.1007/s10508-014-0285-3

29. Gyngell C, Coghill D and Payne J, 'You might have heard ADHD risks being over-diagnosed. Here's why that's not the case', *The Conversation*, 28 June 2023. https://theconversation.com/you-might-have-heard-adhd-risks-being-over-diagnosed-heres-why-thats-not-the-case-208581

30. Myths and Misunderstandings, CHADD, accessed September 2024. https://chadd.org/about-adhd/myths-and-misunderstandings

31. Lockett E, 'Common signs of Attention Deficit Hyperactivity Disorder (ADHD)', *Healthline*, updated March 2022. https://www.healthline.com/health/adhd/signs#takeaway

32. Rogers DC, Dittner AJ, Rimes KA and Chalder T, 'Fatigue in an adult attention deficit hyperactivity disorder population: A trans-diagnostic approach', *Br J Clin Psychol*, vol. 56, pages 33–52, 2017. https://doi.org/10.1111/bjc.12119

33. 'What I would never trade away', *ADDitude*, July 2022 https://www.additudemag.com/slideshows/positives-of-adhd

34. *Diagnostic and Statistical Manual of Mental Disorders* (5th ed.), American Psychiatric Association, 2013. https://doi.org/10.1176/appi.books.9780890425596

35. ICD-11 for Mortality and Morbidity Statistics: Attention deficit hyperactivity disorder, International Statistical Classification of Diseases and Related Health Problems, 11th Revision, World Health Organization, 2024. https://icd.who.int/browse/2024-01/mms/en#821852937

ADHD UNPACKED

36. Stein DJ, Szatmari P, Gaebel W et al, 'Mental, behavioral and neurodevelopmental disorders in the ICD-11: an international perspective on key changes and controversies', *BMC Medicine*, vol. 18(1), article 21, 2020. https://doi.org/10.1186/s12916-020-1495-2

37. Adamou M. 'Why it makes economic sense to treat adult ADHD', *ADHD in Practice*, vol. 2 (3), 2010. http://eprints.hud.ac.uk/id/eprint/11294/

38. Ornoy A and Spivak A. 'Cost effectiveness of optimal treatment of ADHD in Israel: a suggestion for national policy', *Health Economics Review*, vol. 9(1), article 24, 2019. https://doi.org/10.1186/s13561-019-0240-z

39. Daley D, Jacobsen RG, Lange A-M et al, 'The economic burden of adult attention deficit hyperactivity disorder: A sibling comparison cost analysis', *European Psychiatry: the Journal of the Association of European Psychiatrists*, vol. 61, pages 41–48, 2019. doi:10.1016/j.eurpsy.2019.06.011

40. 'Updated European Consensus Statement on diagnosis and treatment of adult ADHD', *European Psychiatry*, vol. 56, pages 14–34, 2019. doi: 10.1016/j.eurpsy.2018.11.001 https://pubmed.ncbi.nlm.nih.gov/30453134/

41. Kolevzon A, 'Current trends in the pharmacological treatment of autism spectrum disorders', in *The Neuroscience of Autism Spectrum Disorders*, Elsevier eBook, pages 85–101, 2013. https://doi.org/10.1016/b978-0-12-391924-3.00006-5

42. Zhang L, Yao H, Li L et al, 'Risk of Cardiovascular Diseases Associated With Medications Used in Attention-Deficit/Hyperactivity Disorder: A Systematic Review and Meta-analysis', *JAMA Network Open*, vol. 5(11), page e2243597, 2022. https://doi.org/10.1001/jamanetworkopen.2022.43597

43. 'Attention deficit hyperactivity disorder: diagnosis and management. Maintenance and monitoring', NICE Guideline NG87, National Institute for Health and Care Excellence (NICE), last updated September 2019. https://www.nice.org.uk/guidance/ng87/chapter/Recommendations#-maintenance-and-monitoring

44. Vázquez JC, Martin de la Torre O, López Palomé J and Redolar-Ripoll D, 'Effects of Caffeine Consumption on Attention Deficit Hyperactivity Disorder (ADHD) Treatment: A Systematic Review of Animal Studies.' *Nutrients*, vol. 14(4), page 739, 2022. https://doi.org/10.3390/nu14040739

45. 'Attention deficit hyperactivity disorder: diagnosis and management', Rationale and Impact: Managing ADHD – adults, NICE Guideline NG87, National Institute for Health and Care Excellence (NICE), last updated September 2019. https://www.nice.org.uk/guidance/ng87/chapter/Rationale-and-impact#managing-adhd-adults

46. López P, Torrente F, Ciapponi A et al, 'Cognitive-behavioural interventions for attention deficit hyperactivity disorder (ADHD) in adults', *Cochrane Database of Systematic Reviews*, issue 3, 2018. https://doi.org/10.1002/14651858.cd010840.pub2

47. Yao L, Guyatt GH and Djulbegovic B, 'Can we trust strong recommendations based on low quality evidence?', *British Medical Journal*, volume 375, n2833, 2021. https://doi.org/10.1136/bmj.n2833

REFERENCES

48. 'The Professional Charter for Coaching, Mentoring and Supervision of Coaches, Mentors and Supervisors', European Economic and Social Council, European Commission, accessed September 2024. https://www.eesc.europa.eu/en/policies/policy-areas/enterprise/database-self-and-co-regulation-initiatives/150

49. 'New Directions on ADHD and Better Sleep', CHADD, accessed September 2024. https://chadd.org/adhd-weekly/new-directions-on-adhd-and-better-sleep/

50. 'Trust levels towards pharma industry, by country 2021', Statista, 2023 https://www.statista.com/statistics/1071584/trust-levels-towards-pharma-sector-in-select-countries

51. Lee CSC, Ma M-T, Ho HY et al, 'The Effectiveness of Mindfulness-Based Intervention in Attention on Individuals with ADHD: A Systematic Review', *Hong Kong Journal of Occupational Therapy*, vol. 30(1), pages 33–41, 2017. https://doi.org/10.1016/j.hkjot.2017.05.001

52. Seladi-Schulman J, 'What to know about Brillia, a homeopathic product', *Healthline*, 2022. https://www.healthline.com/health/migraine/brillia#-does-it-work.

53. Koch K, McLean J, Segev R et al. 'How much the eye tells the brain', *Curr Biol*, vol. 16(14), pages 1428–34, 2006. doi: 10.1016/j.cub.2006.05.056.

54. Furukawa E, Bado P, Da Costa R et al, 'Reward modality modulates striatal responses to reward anticipation in ADHD: Effects of affiliative and food stimuli', *Psychiatry Research: Neuroimaging*, vol. 327, page 111561, 2022. https://doi.org/10.1016/j.pscychresns.2022.111561

55. Ströhle A, Stoy M, Wrase J et al, 'Reward anticipation and outcomes in adult males with attention-deficit/hyperactivity disorder', *NeuroImage*, vol. 39(3), pages 966–972, 2008. https://doi.org/10.1016/j.neuroimage.2007.09.044

56. Plichta MM and Scheres A, 'Ventral-striatal responsiveness during reward anticipation in ADHD and its relation to trait impulsivity in the healthy population: a meta-analytic review of the fMRI literature', *Neuroscience and Biobehavioral Reviews*, vol. 38, pages 125–34, 2014. doi: 10.1016/j.neubiorev.2013.07.012

57. Paloyelis Y, Mehta MA, Faraone SV et al, 'Striatal sensitivity during reward processing in attention-deficit/hyperactivity disorder', *J Am Acad Child Adolesc Psychiatry*, vol. 51(7), pages 722–732.e9, 2012. doi: 10.1016/j.jaac.2012.05.006.

58. Anselme P and Robinson MJ, 'What motivates gambling behavior? Insight into dopamine's role', *Frontiers in Behavioral Neuroscience*, vol. 7, page 182, 2013. https://doi.org/10.3389/fnbeh.2013.00182

59. Lewis RG, Florio E, Punzo D and Borrelli E, 'The Brain's Reward System in Health and Disease', *Advances in Experimental Medicine and Biology*, vol. 1344, pages 57–69, 2021. https://doi.org/10.1007/978-3-030-81147-1_4

60. Furukawa E, Alsop B, Alves H et al, 'Disrupted waiting behavior in ADHD: exploring the impact of reward availability and predictive

cues', *Child Neuropsychology*, vol. 29(1), pages 76–95, 2023. doi: 10.1080/09297049.2022.2068518

61. Skalski S, Pochwatko G and Balas R, 'Impact of Motivation on Selected Aspects of Attention in Children with ADHD', *Child Psychiatry and Human Development*, vol. 52(1), page 190, 2021. doi: 10.1007/s10578-020-01092-4.

62. Morsink S, Van der Oord S, Antrop I et al, 'Studying Motivation in ADHD: The Role of Internal Motives and the Relevance of Self Determination Theory', *Journal of Attention Disorders*, vol. 26(8), pages 1139–1158, 2022 doi: 10.1177/10870547211050948.

63. Emotion. *APA Dictionary of Psychology*. https://dictionary.apa.org/emotion, updated April 2018.

64. Cullen, K, 'Suppressing emotions can harm you – here's what to do instead', *Psychology Today*, posted December 2022. https://www.psychologytoday.com/intl/blog/the-truth-about-exercise-addiction/202212/suppressing-emotions-can-harm-you-heres-what-to-do

65. Rydzewska M, Zaorska J and Jakubczyk A, 'The regulation of emotions and problematic alcohol use: a review of literature', *Alkoholizm I Narkomania*, vol. 36(2), pages 113–140, 2023. https://doi.org/10.5114/ain.2023.132441

66. Barkley RA, DuPaul GJ and McMurray MB, 'Comprehensive evaluation of attention deficit disorder with and without hyperactivity as defined by research criteria', *Journal of Consulting and Clinical Psychology*, vol. 58(6), pages 775–789, 1990. https://doi.org/10.1037/0022-006X.58.6.775

67. Stenseng F, Belsky J, Skalicka V and Wichstrøm L, 'Peer Rejection and Attention Deficit Hyperactivity Disorder Symptoms: Reciprocal Relations Through Ages 4, 6, and 8', *Child Development*, 2015; vol. 87(2), pages 365–73. doi: 10.1111/cdev.12471

68. Downey G and Feldman SI, 'Implications of rejection sensitivity for intimate relationships', *Journal of Personality and Social Psychology*, vol. 70(6), pages 1327–1343, 1996. doi:10.1037/0022-3514.70.6.1327.

69. Salehinejad MA, Ghanavati E, Rashid MHA and Nitsche MA, 'Hot and cold executive functions in the brain: A prefrontal-cingular network', *Brain and Neuroscience Advances*, vol. 5, 2021. https://doi.org/10.1177/23982128211007769

70. Ortega R, López V, Carrasco X et al, 'Neurocognitive mechanisms underlying working memory encoding and retrieval in Attention-Deficit/Hyperactivity Disorder', *Sci Rep*, vol. 10, article 7771, 2020. https://doi.org/10.1038/s41598-020-64678-x

71. Bálint S, Bitter I, and Czobor P, 'A kognitív rugalmasság neurobiológiai korrelátumainak vizsgálata ADHD-ban Irodalmi áttekintés [Neurobiological correlates of cognitive flexibility in ADHD – A systematic review of the literature]', *Psychiatria Hungarica : A Magyar Pszichiatriai Tarsasag tudomanyos folyoirata*, vol. 30(4), pages 363–71, 2015. https://pubmed.ncbi.nlm.nih.gov/26771696/

REFERENCES

72. Umbach G, Kantak P, Jacobs J et al, 'Time cells in the human hippocampus and entorhinal cortex support episodic memory', *Proceedings of the National Academy of Sciences of the United States of America*, vol. 117(45), pages 28463–28474, 2020. https://doi.org/10.1073/pnas.2013250117

73. Mette C, 'Time Perception in Adult ADHD: Findings from a Decade—A Review', *International Journal of Environmental Research and Public Health/International Journal of Environmental Research and Public Health*, vol. 20(4), page 3098, 2023. https://doi.org/10.3390/ijerph20043098

74. Ptacek R, Weissenberger S, Braaten E et al, 'Clinical Implications of the Perception of Time in Attention Deficit Hyperactivity Disorder (ADHD): A Review', *Medical Science Monitor: International Medical Journal of Experimental and Clinical Research*, vol. 25, pages 3918–3924, 2019. https://doi.org/10.12659/MSM.914225

75. Marx I, Cortese, S, Koelch, MG and Hacker T, 'Meta-analysis: Altered perceptual timing abilities in Attention-Deficit/Hyperactivity Disorder', *Journal of the American Academy of Child and Adolescent Psychiatry*, vol. 61(7), pages 866–880, 2021. https://doi.org/10.1016/j.jaac.2021.12.004

76. Noreika V, Falter CM and Rubia K, 'Timing deficits in attention-deficit/hyperactivity disorder (ADHD): Evidence from neurocognitive and neuroimaging studies', *Neuropsychologia*, vol. 51(2), pages 235–266, 2013. https://doi.org/10.1016/j.neuropsychologia.2012.09.036

77. Dekkers TJ, Popma A, Van Rentergem JAA et al, 'Risky decision making in Attention-Deficit/Hyperactivity Disorder: A meta-regression analysis', *Clinical Psychology Review*, vol 45, pages 1–16, 2016. https://doi.org/10.1016/j.cpr.2016.03.001

78. Dekkers TJ, Popma A, Van Rentergem JAA et al, 'Risky decision making in Attention-Deficit/Hyperactivity Disorder: A meta-regression analysis', *Clinical Psychology Review*, vol 45, pages 1–16, 2016. https://doi.org/10.1016/j.cpr.2016.03.001

79. Moyá J, Stringaris AK, Asherson P et al, 'The impact of persisting hyperactivity on social relationships: a community-based, controlled 20-year follow-up study', *Journal of Attention Disorders*, vol. 18(1), pages 52–60, 2014. doi: 10.1177/1087054712436876.

80. Glass K, Flory K and Hankin BL, 'Symptoms of ADHD and close friendships in adolescence', *Journal of Attention Disorders*, vol. 16(5), pages 406–417, 2010. https://doi.org/10.1177/1087054710390865

81. Spender K, Chen YR, Wilkes-Gillan S et al, 'The friendships of children and youth with attention-deficit hyperactivity disorder: A systematic review', *PloS one*, vol. 18(8), page e0289539, 2023. https://doi.org/10.1371/journal.pone.0289539

82. Kessler RC, Adler L, Barkley R et al, 'The prevalence and correlates of adult ADHD in the United States: results from the National Comorbidity Survey Replication', *The American Journal of Psychiatry*, vol. 163(4), pages 716–723, 2006. https://doi.org/10.1176/ajp.2006.163.4.716

83. Jakobsson SS, Van Zalk N, Granander SW et al, 'The Relationship Betwe-

en Social Anxiety Disorder and ADHD in Adolescents and Adults: A Systematic Review', *J Atten Disord*, vol. 28(9), pages 1299–1319, 2024. doi: 10.1177/10870547241247448.

84. Kendall J, 'Sibling accounts of Attention Deficit Hyperactivity Disorder (ADHD)', *Family Process*, vol. 38(1), pages 117–136, 1999. https://doi.org/10.1111/j.1545-5300.1999.00117.x

85. Faraone SV, Banaschewski T, Coghill D et al, 'The World Federation of ADHD International Consensus Statement: 208 Evidence-based conclusions about the disorder', *Neuroscience and Biobehavioral Reviews*, vol. 128, pages 789–818, 2021. https://doi.org/10.1016/j.neubiorev.2021.01.022

86. Montejo JE, Durán M, Del Mar Martínez M et al, 'Family functioning and parental bonding during childhood in adults diagnosed with ADHD', *Journal of Attention Disorders*, vol. 23(1), pages 57–64, 2015. https://doi.org/10.1177/1087054715596578

87. McKee TE, Harvey E, Danforth JS et al, 'The relation between parental coping styles and parent-child interactions before and after treatment for children with ADHD and oppositional behavior', *Journal of Clinical Child and Adolescent Psychology*, vol. 33(1), pages 158–168, 2004. https://doi.org/10.1207/s15374424jccp3301_15

88. Küpper T, Haavik J, Drexler H et al, 'The negative impact of attention-deficit/hyperactivity disorder on occupational health in adults and adolescents', *Int Arch Occup Environ Health*, vol. 85, pages 837–847, 2012. https://doi.org/10.1007/s00420-012-0794-0

89. Beaton DM, Sirois F and Milne E, 'Experiences of criticism in adults with ADHD: A qualitative study', *PloS One*, vol. 17(2), page e0263366, 2022b. https://doi.org/10.1371/journal.pone.0263366

90. Lopez V, 'So apparently a quarter of single people aren't interested in monogamy', *Cosmopolitan*, published March 2022. https://www.cosmopolitan.com/sex-love/a39430353/relationship-statistics-2022/

91. Levine H, 'How ADHD can affect your marriage', *WebMD*, published July 2022. https://www.webmd.com/add-adhd/adult-adhd-marriage

92. Young S, Klassen LJ, Reitmeier SD et al, 'Let's Talk about Sex... and ADHD: Findings from an Anonymous Online Survey', *International Journal of Environmental Research and Public Health*, vol. 20(3), page 2037, 2023. https://doi.org/10.3390/ijerph20032037

93. Skalski S, Pochwatko G and Balas R, 'Impact of Motivation on Selected Aspects of Attention in Children with ADHD', *Child Psychiatry and Human Development*, vol. 52(4), pages 586–595, 2021. https://doi.org/10.1007/s10578-020-01042-0

94. Habbert R and Schroeder J, 'To build efficacy, eat the frog first: People misunderstand how the difficulty-ordering of tasks influences efficacy', *Journal of Experimental Social Psychology*, vol. 91, page 104032, 2020. https://doi.org/10.1016/j.jesp.2020.104032

95. ICD-11 for Mortality and Morbidity Statistics, World Health Organization (WHO), https://icd.who.int/browse/2024-01/mms/en#821852937

REFERENCES

96. Oguchi M, Takahashi T, Nitta Y and Kumano H, 'The moderating effect of Attention-Deficit Hyperactivity Disorder symptoms on the relationship between procrastination and internalizing symptoms in the general adult population', *Frontiers in Psychology*, vol. 12, page 708579, 2021. doi: 10.3389/fpsyg.2021.708579

97. Turgeman RN and Pollak Y, 'Using the temporal motivation theory to explain the relation between ADHD and procrastination', *Australian Psychologist*, vol. 58(6), pages 448–456, 2023 https://doi.org/10.1080/00050067.2023.2218540

98. Sirois FM, Molnar DS and Hirsch JK, 'A Meta–Analytic and Conceptual Update on the Associations between Procrastination and Multidimensional Perfectionism', *European Journal of Personality*, vol. 31(2), pages 137–159, 2017. https://doi.org/10.1002/per.2098

99. Müller V, Mellor D and Piko BF, 'How to procrastinate productively with ADHD: A study of smartphone use, depression, and other academic variables among university students with ADHD symptoms', *Journal of Attention Disorders*, vol. 27(9), pages 951–959, 2023. https://doi.org/10.1177/10870547231171724

100. Strohmeier CW, Rosenfield B, DiTomasso RA and Ramsay JR, 'Assessment of the relationship between self-reported cognitive distortions and adult ADHD, anxiety, depression, and hopelessness', *Psychiatry Res*, vol. 238, pages 153–158, 2016. doi: 10.1016/j.psychres.2016.02.034.

101. Kessler RC, Lane M, Stang PE and Van Brunt DL, 'The prevalence and workplace costs of adult attention deficit hyperactivity disorder in a large manufacturing firm', *Psychol Med*, vol. 39(1), pages 137–47, 2009. doi: 10.1017/S0033291708003309.

102. Hilton MF, Scuffham PA, Sheridan JD et al. 'The Association Between Mental Disorders and Productivity in Treated and Untreated Employees', *Journal of Occupational and Environmental Medicine* vol. 51(9), pages 996–1003, 2009. doi: 10.1097/JOM.0b013e3181b2ea30

103. Brattberg G, 'PTSD and ADHD: Underlying factors in many cases of burnout', *Stress and Health*, vol. 22(5), pages 305–313, 2006. https://doi.org/10.1002/smi.1112

104. Doshi JA, Hodgkins P, Kahle J et al, 'Economic impact of childhood and adult attention-deficit/hyperactivity disorder in the United States', *J Am Acad Child Adolesc Psychiatry*, vol. 51(10), pages 990–1002.e2, 2012. doi: 10.1016/j.jaac.2012.07.008.

105. Katzman MA, Bilkey TS, Chokka PR et al, 'Adult ADHD and comorbid disorders: clinical implications of a dimensional approach', *BMC Psychiatry*, vol. 17(1), page 302, 2017. https://doi.org/10.1186/s12888-017-1463-3

106. 'ADHD and co-occurring conditions', CHADD, accessed September 2024. https://chadd.org/about-adhd/co-occuring-conditions/

107. 'What else you got? The co-existing conditions of adult ADHD', *Focus On Adult ADHD Magazine*, accessed September 2024. https://focusmag.uk/what-else-you-got-the-co-existing-conditions-of-adult-adhd/

ADHD UNPACKED

108. Rietz ED, Brikell I, Butwicka A et al, 'Mapping phenotypic and aetiological associations between ADHD and physical conditions in adulthood in Sweden: a genetically informed register study', *The Lancet Psychiatry*, vol. 8(9), pages 774–783, 2021. doi: https://doi.org/10.1016/S2215-0366(21)00171-1.

109. Kraut AA, Langner I, Lindemann C et al, 'Comorbidities in ADHD children treated with methylphenidate: a database study', *BMC Psychiatry*, vol. 13(1), page 11, 2013. https://doi.org/10.1186/1471-244x-13-11

110. Migueis DP, Lopes MC, Casella E et al, 'Attention deficit hyperactivity disorder and restless leg syndrome across the lifespan: A systematic review and meta-analysis', *Sleep Medicine Reviews*, vol. 69, page 101770, 2023. https://doi.org/10.1016/j.smrv.2023.101770

111. Glans M, Thelin N, Humble MB et al. 'Association between adult attention-deficit hyperactivity disorder and generalised joint hypermobility: A cross-sectional case control comparison', *Journal of Psychiatric Research*, vol. 143, pages 334–340, 2021 doi: 10.1016/j.jpsychires.2021.07.006.

112. Doğan ŞK, Taner Y and Evcik D, 'Benign joint hypermobility syndrome in patients with attention deficit/hyperactivity disorders', *Turkish Journal of Rheumatology*, vol. 26(3), pages 187–192, 2011. doi: https://doi.org/10.5606/tjr.2011.029.

113. Cederlöf M, Larsson H, Lichtenstein P et al, 'Nationwide population-based cohort study of psychiatric disorders in individuals with Ehlers–Danlos syndrome or hypermobility syndrome and their siblings', *BMC Psychiatry*, vol. 16, page 207, 2016. https://doi.org/10.1186/s12888-016-0922-6

114. Termine C, Luoni C, Fontolan S et al, 'Impact of co-morbid attention-deficit and hyperactivity disorder on cognitive function in male children with Tourette syndrome: A controlled study', *Psychiatry Research*, vol. 243, pages 263–267, 2016 https://doi.org/10.1016/j.psychres.2016.06.048

115. Becker SP, 'ADHD and sleep: recent advances and future directions', *Current Opinion in Psychology*, vol. 34, pages 50–56, 2020. https://doi.org/10.1016/j.copsyc.2019.09.006

116. Taurines R, Schmitt J, Renner T et al, 'Developmental comorbidity in attention-deficit/hyperactivity disorder', *Attention Deficit and Hyperactivity Disorders*, vol. 2(4), pages 267–289, 2010. https://doi.org/10.1007/s12402-010-0040-0

117. Taurines R, Schmitt J, Renner T et al, 'Developmental comorbidity in attention-deficit/hyperactivity disorder', *Attention deficit and hyperactivity disorders*, vol. 2(4), pages 267–289, 2010. https://doi.org/10.1007/s12402-010-0040-0

118. *The ADHD Adults Podcast.* https://theadhdadults.uk

Acknowledgements

We would explicitly like to acknowledge those family members and friends who have been incredibly supportive (you know who you are). A notable mention to some incredible people, including (but not limited to) Jack, Nick, Pat (DJ Sessionz), Kirsty, Maria, Eric, Darren, Mireille, Laura (both), Robin and a huge thanks to Anthony and Ros at the wonderful Aston University. If we forgot anyone, oh god that is RSD and we are incredibly sorry.

A Note on the Authors

James Brown and Alex Conner are the co-hosts and founders of the hit ADHD podcast, *The ADHD Adults*. They are both visiting Professors at the fantastic Aston University in Birmingham. James is a scientific researcher and journalist who has been featured on the BBC, ITV, Channel 4, iNews, Forbes and News24. Alex is an academic, coach, journalist and science communicator who has been featured in *Medical News Today*, *News24* and the *Independent*. Both James and Alex have ADHD and were diagnsoed as adults. They are also the founders of the award-winning charity, ADHDadultUK.